# How Cancer Cured My Broken Soul

## A terrifying, raw, and side-splitting tale of one woman's breast cancer journey

## A Memoir

## Nicole L. Czarnomski

**How Cancer Cured My Broken Soul**

Printed in the United States of America

First Printing: April, 2020

ISBN-978-1-661-77171-3

"When something bad happens you have three choices. You can either let it define you, let is destroy you, or you can let it strengthen you."

~ Dr. Seuss

Nicole L. Czarnomski
thewhisperingpen.com

Cover by Laura Drew
lauradrewdesign.com

Edited by Allison Roe
@allison.roe01

Formatting by Beth M. Anderson
womenofwords.com

Nicole L. Czarnomski

# TABLE OF CONTENTS

Nicole L. Czarnomski

# Introduction

Monday, July 3, 2017. The day before my eighth wedding anniversary I was diagnosed with breast cancer. I walked into the appointment alone believing I could handle anything the doctor had to say. I was wrong. The diagnosis left me speechless and inconsolable. I cried walking out of the hospital doors, I cried sitting in the car calling my mother and my husband. I cried the entire car ride to my house, and then sobbed as I fell into my husband's arms at home.

Nothing can prepare a person for a cancer diagnosis. Through it, I found my inner strength, strength I didn't know I possessed. I also found that I am loved more than I could have ever imagined, and that humor is my saving grace.

Writing this book started off as catharsis, but soon blossomed into a means of helping others. My cancer journey taught me more about myself and more about life than anything else I've experienced. Whether you are on this path yourself or you have a friend or family member diagnosed with breast cancer, this book is about overcoming adversity and finding a little humor in seemingly insurmountable challenges. It's about learning to love yourself, celebrating your flaws, and about learning to smile. Always.

# Part 1: The Diagnosis

# Dimples Are Supposed to be Cute

For an entire month, I thought it was a cute dimple. But the dimple wasn't on my face; it was on my right breast.

I hemmed and hawed over making the call. I thought perhaps a new deodorant had irritated a lymph node. I kept looking at the dimple and finally scouted the area with a self-breast exam. A lump. Solid and smooth, it rolled from side to side between my fingers as I checked myself. Damn.

I changed back to my usual deodorant and left it alone for another couple of weeks. I have no family history of breast cancer; it was clearly nothing.

Days passed and I couldn't stop thinking about the dimple and the lump in my right breast. I made the appointment. Five days before my family went on vacation to celebrate my father's retirement, my physician performed a breast exam and concluded the lump was non-worrisome. At my request, she ordered a mammogram and ultrasound. She recommended the ultrasound because the lump was in a weird spot (the upper part of my right breast near my armpit). The mammogram might not catch it well enough on its own. I left the exam feeling optimistic.

Friday, June 23, 2017. Back from vacation, it was time for my radiology appointment. I sat in a waiting room clothed from the waist down, covered on top with only a dusty rose-colored gown that tied in the front. I stared at the warm, earth-toned walls in the waiting area. Fixer Upper played on the television, and I got lost watching the perfect lives of Chip and Joanna as they redesigned and renovated a sad looking old home.

I was called in for the first part of my procedure—the mammogram. The young woman doing the procedure was short with dark, almost black hair. Her nose was pierced with a tiny stud; it reminded me of the one I had gotten back in 2000 when I moved to Colorado. I was a free spirit—an artist. I wanted to stand out from the crowd. When my mom saw it for the first time, she called it a fixture. I felt rebellious and cool. Ten years later, I was bored of the tiny stud. I took it out and was left with a tiny spot where the stud once lived. Now I was just a girl who used to have a nose stud. The spot which is still on my nose reminds me of my once cool, art school days.

The mammogram was an invasive procedure. I was happy to have a woman aligning my breast in the towering machine that flattened poor Righty like a sheet of paper.

As she snapped the image, she told me to hold my breath. This was more challenging than the mashing of my breast—I felt like I was suffocating. Or drowning. Help me, I whispered to myself as I held my breath. I was hoping there wouldn't be lines printed on my boobs like corrugated cardboard when it was over.

The placement of the lump made it difficult for her to get the perfect image, just as my physician predicted. Lucky me. She took picture after picture after picture hoping for the perfect image. After she finally got what she needed, I returned to the waiting room until it was time for the ultrasound.

The waiting room was void of people but filled with endless yammering from television commercials. As the commercials droned on, I heard voices coming down the stairwell from the lobby upstairs. I was in a perfect position to see who was coming down the steps, and they could see me. I heard a male's voice and hoped it was a doctor because I was still cloaked in the dusty rose-colored gown.

To my surprise, the voice came from a silver-haired, elderly man. He didn't look my direction, but I knew exactly who he was. He was a resident at a senior living community where I worked. I saw him almost every day. As if this procedure wasn't difficult enough, now I worried news would spread throughout the campus about getting my boobs checked. Gossip spreads faster at a senior living community than it does at a high school.

Quickly, I darted across the room to a different sofa, one that blocked the view of anyone coming down the stairs. I hoped my game of musical chairs would keep my secret safe. Maybe I could just melt into the faux leather sofa and wait for my next procedure in anonymity.

Thankfully, I didn't have to wait long before the ultrasound technician came to get me. She took me to a large room, bigger than the master bedroom in my home. There were two rows of cabinets extending the entire length of the wall, one high and one low. There was a countertop between them that held a few decorative pieces of art and some paperwork I assumed was mine. In the middle of the room there was a large, adjustable bed with a computer monitor next to it. I lay on the bed with my boobs exposed, focusing on the large panel of landscape images on the ceiling. There was a river flowing over a bed of smooth looking rocks, trees, orange flowers and other nature scenes. I wondered how these images could comfort anyone at a time like this.

The technician pushed and probed on the lump and dove farther into my armpit. What the hell? I thought. The lump was in my breast not my armpit. The technician agreed, saying she saw the same thing I was feeling, but she also felt another lump in my armpit.

The ultrasound technician and the breast care coordinator started whispering to each other. The technician's brow furrowed as she looked at the monitor. She dug deeper and deeper into the hollows of my right arm. The technician whispered, "Do you see both masses?" The coordinator responded with a whisper "yes" and suggested they show the radiologist.

From this invasive procedure, I discovered my breast tissue was dense, which made it difficult to find anything. The technician described it as a snowstorm. She said cancer tumors are difficult to find in dense tissue because they resemble snowballs. When looking at the ultrasound, it was like trying to find a snowball in a snowstorm. She didn't come out and say I had tumors, but the whispers and concerned faces told me something wasn't right.

When the coordinator returned, she said the radiologist believed there were two lumps. What? How could that be? My stomach burned, and my gut spiraled like someone was wringing out a wet rag. Before leaving, they set me up with a biopsy appointment for the following Tuesday. They explained the procedure to me: first, the breast would be numbed. Then a large needle with a coring mechanism would pierce the skin, find the lumps, and pull out tissue in each of the lumps.

Let the fun begin.

The following week, I returned to the doctor's office. This time I went immediately to the chair in the far corner, hidden from the stairwell. There was one other woman in the waiting room and she was wearing the same dusty rose-colored gown I was wearing. She was called first; moments later I was called back to the same room I was in last week.

The radiologist started the biopsy by numbing the area around the dimple. Thankfully, I couldn't see the needle; needles make me woozy. The biopsy wasn't painful, but the machine made unnerving sounds. I could feel pressure against my breast, and then a clicking noise that sounded like an old price sticker machine. Then there was a whirring noise, and I assumed it was the drill digging deeper into the skin tissue. The radiologist wiggled the needle from side to side and I wondered how big the hole in my breast was getting. He dug deeper and peered up at the monitor. Once he found the snowball-looking mass floating around in the tissue, he pulled out a sample. He withdrew so many samples I stopped counting.

When the biopsy was finished, the nurse applied quarter inch medical tape over the entry point in a star pattern and covered it with a Band-Aid. They told me not to shower or do aerobic activity for 24 hours. The bandage was supposed to remain in place for four to five days. I hated the thought of not exercising because it kept me sane, sometimes more than writing in my journal.

While waiting for the results, the biopsy site turned multiple shades of dark purple. It was tender to the touch, but not sore enough for painkillers. The tape stayed in place until I went running 48 hours after the procedure. The movement of my arm rubbed on the tape and created a welt that felt like a rug burn, pulling the tape off. The salty sweat burned the raw skin around the wound. As if that wasn't painful enough, it was time for bomb number one.

Bomb number one dropped on July 3, at my appointment with the general surgeon. I walked into the waiting room and checked in. I sat on another leather chair that felt more like plastic than leather. I looked directly down a hallway leading to the doctors' offices. The sign above said Urology. Hmmm, nothing wrong with my kidneys or bladder. Or wait, was there? My heart fluttered; was there more to the lumps found in my breast?

A woman stood at the end of the hall and called me by my first name. I wondered if she was afraid to pronounce Czarnomski or was it for privacy reasons. She walked me to a sterile looking room. The fluorescent lights were so bright I felt like I needed to smother my body in sunscreen. The walls were pale green I assumed to evoke calmness and serenity, although that was far from what I felt. She took my blood pressure and temperature, and before leaving, asked me to put on a gown.

The damn cover-up was ridiculous! There were six random strings and none of them lined up. I could always get undressed and robed before the doctor arrived, but this time the surgeon beat me. I swaddled the wrap around me and sat down. He introduced himself and shook my hand, dismissing my confusion with the wrap.

My surgeon was an Indian man with a thick accent. His lower teeth were mangled together like stalagmites growing from a cave floor. He was dressed in blue hospital scrubs; had he cut into boobs or a bladder earlier today?

"How are you doing?" he asked. I began to say, I will be doing better once I hear… but before I could finish my sentence, his harsh brown eyes looked directly into mine and with no hesitation, he said, "You have breast cancer."

Boom. It felt like a bully from elementary school had punched me in the gut. Color drained from my face. I sat breathless, tears stuck inside, unwilling to come out. This guy had a horrible bedside manner.

"Are you taking hormone replacement pills?" he asked. I scrunched my face and shook my head no.

"Well, birth control pills. Is that considered a hormone replacement?" I asked. He told me to stop taking them for now. The lab was further examining the tissue to see if the cancer was hormone-based.

A few moments later he asked if I was alright. "Do you have someone here with you?" he asked. I said no. Then he started talking and drawing diagrams and explaining my situation. I wanted to engage in the conversation or at least listen and comprehend, but he kept throwing words at me like grenades; I wanted to duck and hide.

Steadying myself with a deep breath, I forced myself to pay attention. There were two small tumors, one was four millimeters and the other 16 millimeters. He said the type of cancer I had was very treatable and the tumors were slow growing. Apparently, many women have this type of breast cancer. There were several options for me. He told me about a lumpectomy with radiation or mastectomy with reconstructive surgery. He felt my best option would be a double mastectomy because of my dense breast tissue.

The anxiety was overwhelming. I asked if the radiation would make me lose my hair or make me physically ill. "Don't get ahead of yourself. Radiation is not as invasive as chemotherapy, which creates hair loss and vomiting," he said. Relief at last.

There was a certain solace in knowing the tumors were small and slow growing, but this diagnosis had to be incorrect. There was a mistake. Not me. I couldn't possibly have cancer at age 42. There wasn't a history of breast cancer in my family and taking care of my body was top priority to me. Exercise was a part of my everyday life and I chose fruits and veggies over fried or fatty foods 90 percent of the time. I hadn't touched red meat in decades for goodness sake.

The doctor wanted to examine me, so he had the nurse return while he did it. The tissue paper below me crinkled as I reclined back.

After his exam, he covered me, and I sat up. He asked again if there was someone here with me. "Your husband? Your mother? A friend?"

"No, I don't have anyone here with me," I said, annoyed. I lied and told him I was fine. The nurse patted my back and said it was okay to cry. I don't know why I needed permission, but finally, I let myself cry. I pressed my face into my hands and let the cold, steady stream of tears run down my face and arms.

The tears were the doctor's cue to leave. "Do you have any more questions for me?" he asked. I shook my head and he left. The nurse sat with me for a few more minutes until the breast care coordinator arrived. She brought me a small, brown canvas bag with pink handles. Her voice was gentle and caring. She reminded me that my prognosis looked good because of the type of tumor and its small size, and I began to calm down. I appreciated her empathy, but also wanted to punch her in the face because she wasn't the one with cancer. She pulled out a large medical textbook from the boobie bag. I cringed. A freaking textbook? I wanted real people, real stories. The bag also included a boobie pillow to be used during transportation after any surgeries. The pillow was pink and moon shaped, and I didn't have a clue as to how to use it. There were two small pamphlets, a notebook and an accordion file to fill with all the new information I would be getting in the next several weeks.

After our meeting, my boobie bag comforted me while walking through the waiting room, tears still falling. My make-up melted, and mascara smudges had pooled around my eyes. The receptionist smiled as she said good-bye in her chipper voice. I opened the door and walked the lonely 20 yards to my car. Sitting in the hot car, I wondered who to call first.

The dashboard in my car lit up when I turned the key. A gentle breeze blew through my car drying out the sweat droplets. My first call was to my employer to let them know I wouldn't be coming back to the office today, because I had cancer. (This now seems totally absurd that I called my employer first.) Sobbing uncontrollably, I hung up the phone. "Please wake up," I sobbed to myself. "It's time to wake up and get out of bed," I pleaded.

But this wasn't a dream. The results were not a mistake. This was my reality. I sat in my car another minute waiting, hoping for a phone call from the breast care coordinator apologizing for this horrific mistake. But these results were mine. They were real, and they were final.

My mother was the next person on my call list. She listened quietly as I wept. "We are going to get through this together," she said. Her voice never wavered. But the only thought I had was, my God, I am going to leave all these beautiful people behind, and it will be harder on them because they will have to live with my death.

There was still no fighting the tears and the ugly cry that had taken over me when my husband picked up the phone call from me. His words mimicked my mother's like they had already spoken. We'll get through this together. Another wave of sadness hit me. One deeper than anything I have ever felt. I hadn't made our relationship a priority; instead I was working full-time and picking up freelance writing jobs to grow my byline. My weekends were filled with writing assignments while my weeknights were filled with teaching fitness classes or preparing for 5k and 10k races. My husband was forced to entertain himself. I felt like a terrible wife. Now, I was a terrible wife with cancer.

What would I say on my death bed? I would tell him to find someone else, to remember me, but find someone else to love. I would tell him to find someone who would share a hunting experience with him, someone who loved to ride in boats that go really fast, someone who was a better wife than me.

I sobbed the entire way home despite the positive outlook of the doctor. I felt like there was no hope for a new life after cancer. My doctor drank from the glass that was half full, while I was drinking the dregs at the bottom.

I don't remember eating that night. What I do remember was being unable to breathe because I had cried hysterically for so many hours. Crying made my head congested; it was like suffocation. I couldn't sleep lying down because of the congestion, so I propped my pillow up and fell asleep sitting up. Before I fell into a deep slumber, my body jerked, and I nearly fell out of bed. I rolled over to spoon my husband hoping he knew how much I loved him and hoping I wouldn't suffocate.

# Nothing to Celebrate

The day after my diagnosis, Tuesday, July fourth, was my eighth wedding anniversary. Adlai and I both slept in and didn't know what to say when we finally got out of bed. We were supposed to be doing something fun, something to celebrate eight beautiful years, but I was still in pity party mode. There was nothing to celebrate, just puffy, swollen eyes from all the crying yesterday.

Memories of my life with Adlai drifted in and out as I sat across from him at breakfast. Memories from our wedding day looped in my brain like a movie reel. My parents hosted the big day at their home in Missouri. We only invited 28 people to the event. Immediate family, friends who introduced us, and close friends of the family. I didn't want anything ostentatious. I wasn't a princess, and I was not about to go into debt to pay for a wedding.

The day started off with early morning rain that stopped by 9 a.m. My hairdresser arrived around the same time the precipitation ended. She spiral-curled my shoulder length blonde hair and pulled the sides up with bobby pins. As I put make-up on, Hy-Vee delivered cold cuts, fruit and a wedding cake. My mom's friend, Shelly, offered to help with the food table and had everything ready immediately following the ceremony at 11:00 a.m.

I was jolted back to reality when Adlai asked, "What would you like to do today?"

"What?" I murmured.

"Would you like to go for a bike ride or canoe the back waters of the Mississippi?"

"I suppose a bike ride would be nice. Let's go to Lanesboro," I said. Lanesboro is a charming town in southeastern Minnesota. There

14

are artisan shops selling everything from homemade soaps and lotions to high priced art. The town has bike and kayak rentals and a few small restaurants. There are no chain stores or franchises anywhere, a respite from the rest of the world.

We had ridden the bike path many times before. The well-manicured trail system was surrounded by beautiful deciduous trees and rocky limestone cliff faces. The trail hugged the Root River and cut through a few farms. It was sunny that day and the temperature hovered around 75.

How could such a perfect day be so far from perfect?

On the drive to Lanesboro, I kept my forehead pressed into the window of Adlai's truck watching the cornfields pass by, getting lost in the memory of what was once a beautiful celebration, a day shared with family, friends, and the love of my life. We rode in silence.

When we arrived, we pulled our bikes from the bed of the truck. "It's a beautiful day for a ride," he said looking at the cloudless, blue sky. We biked up the street and found the trail. We rode four and a half miles to Whalan and took a break. We sat in the shade quietly trying to find something to talk about that wouldn't cause me to go into a crying fit. Turns out that finding words for a conversation was like a toddler trying to play Sudoku, so we got back on the bike trail.

The trail was crowded, people on tandems, and parents riding alongside their children. I pushed the pedals down feeling the muscles in my legs burn, burning like my stomach had hours ago after receiving my diagnosis. I wanted to push the cancer out of my system. I pumped my legs harder and harder, the pedals digging into the soles of my tennis shoes. I looked over my shoulder several times to make sure Adlai was behind me. He was only ever a few feet away no matter how hard I pushed, and I knew he was going to stand tall and support me through this entire journey.

We decided to get a snack in Whalan on our return trip. We stopped at the World's Famous Pie place. Adlai picked a peanut butter pie with a chocolate crumbly crust. I went with a scoop of butter pecan ice cream. We sat in a couple of chairs on their sunporch and watched the couples and families riding their bikes. I wasn't much of a conversationalist, so Adlai took control. I heard him talking, but I wasn't listening. Thoughts of cancer dominated my brain space; I didn't have room for talking about the beauty of this day.

On the ride back to Lanesboro, we crossed over a bridge full of teenage girls looking over the edge. It was about a 20-foot drop into the Root River. Cat calls drifted up from below. Adlai and I stopped and looked over the edge. There were about 30 people flopped inside of inflatable yellow inner tubes all linked together. It was like the Party Cove at the Lake of the Ozarks in Missouri. The people below, mostly males, were encouraging the girls to jump off the bridge and into the river. It was upsetting. I wanted to grab the girls' shoulders and shake them, to scream at them, "What are you thinking? You may lose your life jumping off a stupid bridge into water that is way too shallow." I wanted those girls to live a long and healthy life, unlike me who might soon die from cancer.

I couldn't bring myself to say anything, but my heart ached. I wanted to cry, but not on the trail for everyone to see, so I pedaled on hoping our cycling trip would end soon.

When we returned home that night, I fixed a delicious meal: a meatless chicken patty for myself, and a sautéed chicken breast with olive oil and mushrooms for Adlai. Kale and beet greens were the side dishes, and beet brownies for dessert. I tried to make the dinner with love because I didn't know how many more meals I would be preparing. I couldn't shake the feeling of death looming over me, so I focused on making the perfect meal. Unfortunately, my fear, worry, hesitation and anger, was transferred directly into our dinner–Adlai got food poisoning from the chicken. I had cursed our lovely meal. Not only was he ill for two days, he would have to deal with my cancer along with me, who couldn't even cook chicken.

I was a horrible wife.

The following Friday, a mere four days after my diagnosis, the doctor scheduled me for bloodwork, a chest x-ray and an MRI. This time, Adlai was by my side.

I had to fast before this procedure, and I was completely parched by the time the appointment started at 11 a.m. The importance of having Adlai with me soon became evident, as I started crying in the waiting room. I was already sick of crying, and I wasn't even a week in.

A large, wheezing woman walked into the waiting room and sat across from us. I wondered if she had to fast. I wondered if she was just as thirsty as I was. I wondered if she had cancer. I wanted to cry for her.

The phlebotomist called my name, her expression morose like she knew I had cancer. She led me to a small private room. There was an oversized chair, and when I sat down, my feet barely reached the floor. I sat quietly in the chair, my gaze drifting to the other side of the small room. I looked away as she tied the orange rubber tourniquet around my toned bicep. In a despondent tone, she asked about the weather, a poor effort of distraction. I wasn't a child; I could take this needle prick I told myself. "3-2-1 little stick..." Shit! That hurt! I wondered how big the needle was. It was less of a little stick and more like a burning gouge. Maybe my veins were distraught as well. It felt like someone sucked out my insides with a straw and then blew out the contents with such force the gore stuck to the wall. If my body felt pillaged, I was sure my veins were affected too.

I walked out of my room with a small, white, gauze bandage around the gouge. Adlai was sitting alone. The plump, wheezing woman was gone. He noticed the tears running down my cheeks, so he played a cat video on YouTube. I stopped crying, and I started giggling at the kitties chasing their tails, pawing at water dripping from a faucet and play fighting with a mirror. I looked at Adlai and smiled. "Thank you," I said softly. "I love you."

He picked the perfect moment to say, "We're going to get through this. Be strong. I know you have it in you, but you have to be the one to find it."

The x-ray tech arrived moments later. Alex was a petite and happy fellow who looked like he was 18. He took me to an enormous room with a large machine suspended from the ceiling. He showed me to the changing area and asked me to disrobe on the top and stay dressed from the waist down. There were two bluish green gowns sitting in the changing area. One gown tied in back and the other tied in front. I felt a sense of relief when the strings matched; no wardrobe malfunctions for this test.

Alex guided me in front of a large machine. He took four pictures. Front, right side and left side and one to grow on. I stood there and waited as he excused himself to look over the x-rays.

Upon his return, he smiled and told me to get dressed. His happy little face annoyed me. I wondered if he knew my results. Was it worse than breast cancer? Was there more cancer in my lungs? My heart? I wanted him to tell me what he saw, but I decided not to waste my breath; he was there to take the pictures, not analyze them. I dressed and went back to the waiting room.

Nicole L. Czarnomski

I waited for another 15 minutes before the nurse came for the MRI. She explained to Adlai and me that it would be about 40 minutes, but part of the 40 minutes is undressing and dressing and getting situated. She said, "The actual MRI is relatively short. You're in the MRI machine for only 20 minutes or so." I walked with her to the MRI room and undressed again.

Another gown I couldn't tie. What was it with these gowns and mismatched strings? I wondered who the designer was. I stripped down and left my socks and underwear on. Granny panties. Damn. (Note to self, buy cute underwear for occasions like these.)

I came out of the dressing room in my robe with mismatched strings. The MRI tech said, "We need to insert a tube into your arm for the saline injection." My knees buckled. Wasn't one needle stick today enough? The tech had me sit down and asked me twice if I was feeling okay. I told her I was fine but that I wasn't a fan of needles. "Are you sure you are okay?" She said. The room started to spin, and I realized I was not fine. She let me rest for a couple of minutes, long enough for some color to return to my face.

After the catheter was inserted, she handed me two stickers each with a small clear pouch in the middle. They were to be placed on my nipple. The liquid inside the sticker was used so doctors knew the location of the tumors in relation to my nipples. I went back into the dressing room and came out with stickered nipples. Perhaps the name of a new drink?

At this point, it was time for the MRI. The tech had me lay face down on the small mobile bed. I felt like I was on the massage table. Wouldn't that be nice? My breasts were stuck in two little areas with padding on the sides—for comfort, I guess. They gave me a pair of large yellow headphones that made me feel like I should be on the shooting range popping off rounds of a bolt action .30-.06 rather than in

19

an MRI machine. Before entering, she asked me what type of music I wanted to listen to. "Classic rock," I said without hesitation.

Once situated on the mobile platform, the music started, and I felt the bed moving into the big machine. My heart was pumping louder than the music. As the bed moved, the emergency button's cord was stuck on something. It was about to be yanked from my hand; my panic button gone forever. I squeezed the button with such force I thought it may crumble to ashes in my palm.

"Uh, hey! This thing is stuck," I shouted.

"Oh, sorry my bad," she said with a hint of embarrassment. The MRI tech unhooked the cord from the side of the table; disaster averted.

The next disaster was my bad. The bed started moving again and the music was still pumping. I squeezed the emergency button immediately. "Stop. Stop the music," I shouted at her.

"What's wrong? What do you need?" she asked.

"Give me yoga music, meditation music, something calm. Please yoga music! Please, change the music!" I was on the verge of tears. She changed it to classical. It was time for my first MRI. A test that would show my doctors what lurked inside of my chest cavity.

The bed creeped inside the MRI machine, and I pretended I was getting a massage while practicing deep breathing techniques (smell the roses, blow out the candle.) Once inside, unnerving sounds from the machine pulsed in the earphones. Sounds clunked a thunderous roar and the classical music was barely audible, everything was bouncing around in my head. I reminded myself that I only had one job. Lay still. Before long, the thumping stopped, and the bed began to exit the machine.

"The images were clear, Nicole. You did a great job laying still," said the technician. I couldn't help wondering what they saw on the images. Was more bad news on the horizon? I would have to wait until Monday for the results.

At work on Monday, I hibernated in my office, struggling to concentrate on the simplest tasks waiting for a phone call from my surgeon. I felt like a tightrope walker above the Grand Canyon. Every step was slow and unsteady, the canyon waiting to envelop my body and soul. When my phone rang, it shook me from my deepest, darkest thoughts. The appointment was scheduled, and the MRI results were only a few hours away.

Adlai picked me up from work, and we went to the appointment together. When he pulled into the parking lot, I started to cry. "Why are you crying?" he asked. It was moments like these when I wanted to scream, "What the fuck do you think is wrong! I have fucking cancer!" But I didn't. Instead, I let the rivulets of tears dig crevices in my face, and then as fast as the emotions overcame my mind, I let them go. I had to be strong to face the news waiting for me. Inhale. Exhale. Inhale. Exhale.

We walked inside.

The opening remarks were devastating. The surgeon said the MRI detected another spot on the left side along with the two more spots, for a total of four, on the right side. One of the lesions on the right side was where the lymph nodes were located. He ordered another ultrasound.

Before the general surgeon left, he asked if I was thinking about a lumpectomy or double mastectomy. I told him I thought my best option was a double mastectomy with reconstruction. He seemed comforted. "Nicole, if you were my family member, this is what I would recommend for them," he said. It was the first time I felt important to him, not just like another patient in the system.

As I made an appointment for another ultrasound, I could feel the tension at the base of my skull pouring down through my shoulders and back. My muscles ached from stress, and once again, I was waiting to find out if I had more tumors.

During the next ultrasound, the nurse and the technician began whispering again. My palms clenched involuntarily, like a heartbeat. I prepared for the worst. The breast care coordinator went back and forth between me and the radiologist's office; they found another area to look at further down on the right side. My fingernails dug into my palms. I desperately wanted someone to come running into my room yelling you've been punked! I still couldn't shake the feeling that this was all a huge mistake.

I kept counting, one lesion, two lesions, three lesions, four lesions. Every time the technician stopped the probe and dug deeper, I prepared myself for more bad news.

To my surprise, they released me without another biopsy. The mass on the left breast was non-worrisome and they believed there were only two masses on the right side. This was the first good news I had had in over a week! I unclenched my hands and they throbbed with relief. I wanted to celebrate, until I remembered that I still had cancer.

22

# Go Big or Go Home

Adlai and I met with a plastic surgeon on Friday, July 14. It felt like four or five lifetimes had passed since I received my diagnosis, but it had only been 11 days. I found myself in yet another doctor's office, but the plastic surgeon's office had more panache than the others. The walls were a warm cream with a golden accent wall. The love seat in the room fit just one person. It was comforting and cozy, almost too cozy. Adlai had to sit on a stool with wheels because there was no room for him unless he sat on the patient's table or the doctor's chair.

The first nurse I met had a kind smile and a soft voice. She shared her story of breast reconstruction at age 36. There was a history of breast cancer in her family, and she wanted to be proactive. Her decision seemed dramatic. Maybe there was more to her story.

Her voice continued, soft and quiet. I wondered if someone was eavesdropping in the hallway. As she was getting to know Adlai and me, she warned us about the surgeon we were about to meet.

"Your plastic surgeon looks very young, but he has a lot of experience," she said. "He interned at a very prestigious hospital and he does a great job. People love him."

A little red flag started waving in my head as she spoke. Why did she feel compelled to tell us he was young, experienced and well-liked? Did he intern at the Mayo Clinic? Johns Hopkins? Were those the prestigious hospitals? Why wouldn't he stay at either of those? Maybe he wasn't good enough. I let her continue but remained suspicious of the young doctor I was about to meet.

She talked briefly about the procedure but wanted Doogie Howser to do most of that. As she spoke, I joked about taking fat from different places on my body to create a new set of girls. She told me it was likely that my body didn't have enough fat to create the same size

23

C cup that I had. I was in awe of this because when I poked at my belly it seemed like there was plenty to go around.

"Trust me, we can evaluate your tummy, but you are pretty slim," she said. I took that for the win. Something good in all of this. I was slim.

"How 'bout my butt? I've got lots back there," I said half joking, half serious. She said transferring fat from the buttocks was something to review with the surgeon.

"Super!" I said. "A butt tuck too!" Her face was indifferent. I guess she didn't appreciate my humor.

Before she left, she had me put on a tattered gown that tied in the front. The binding around the edges was falling off and the threads were shredding. It seemed odd to have a stylish doctor's office, but ratty, faded robes for patients. I guess I was expecting some posh, pristine white terry cloth robe found at a spa or retreat center. While fumbling with the strings I wondered how a person with a master's degree struggled to tie four strings on a robe for some privacy.

It was short and fell to my waist just below my belly button, and again, the damn ties would not line up. It didn't matter because I had to open my gown for pictures. I watched Adlai look away when I opened the gown. I was embarrassed. My entire body flushed with heat, tiny beads of perspiration dotted my forehead, and sweat pumped out from my armpits. The nurse took images from the front and both right and left sides. She left the camera on the desk for the plastic surgeon in case he needed additional photos.

When he entered the small room, things went from cozy to claustrophobic. And, oh boy, he looked YOUNG. What the hell? He was extremely handsome too. He reminded me of Pej Vahdat who plays Arastoo on the hit T.V. show "Bones." He was soft spoken with a kind demeanor. I wondered if the criterion to work in a plastic surgeon's office was to have a soft voice. Is that a learned thing, like a commoner learning the proper etiquette to become a princess? Was it a natural thing? Was my DNA deficient in whispering?

He tried to establish rapport as he whispered to all of us. I don't remember anything he said because I couldn't get past his good looks. His eyes were dark and charismatic. His dark hair was wavy with a hint of gel. He had smooth olive skin, not a wrinkle in sight. I pictured him driving around town in a sporty red convertible. Not a late model Porsche, since he was young and probably paying off student loans, but a pre-owned Lexus.

He wanted to measure and examine my girls. I inhaled as if it were my last breath. I could feel the breath all the way to my toes, and then I exhaled. This gorgeous doctor was touching my tatas while my husband was watching. It was like an embarrassing threesome only my husband didn't get to participate. My whole body flushed red. To make matters worse, I said to the hot doctor, "I am so nervous I am sweating under my armpits." I felt like Molly Shannon's Catholic school girl character on Saturday Night Live. He reassured me that it was okay to be nervous.

My gown lay open for the entire world to see my middle-aged, slightly saggy boobs. He measured from the middle of my clavicle down to each nipple and then from nipple to nipple. He said the breast symmetry was very rare. I was furious; how could my perfectly symmetrical ladies have cancer? It didn't seem fair to have the perfect breast triangle and to have them sliced off it because of cancer.

"The nurse said you were interested in transferring fat from your tummy," said the doctor. "Why don't you undo your trousers and open them up. Let me take a look." The room started spinning and I felt a sweat droplet run down from my right armpit. I hoped the gown would absorb the perspiration.

I lowered my pinstriped trousers and of course I had on dark gray granny panties. He looked at the scar resting on my bikini line with a blank expression. I had an ovarian cyst the size of a small grapefruit removed in my early 20s. At that time, the general surgeon put me back together with staples. The scar is harsh and hidden by the shadow of tiny layer of fat that bulges over the long, lost incision. He didn't remark at the harsh reconstruction, but he determined there wasn't adequate fat on my tummy for a C cup. His best guess was an A cup.

Then, he asked me to turn around and drop my trousers. "Are you serious?" I asked like I forgot it was me who asked about this very procedure 10 minutes ago.

"Yes," he said, "if you want me to evaluate the tissue for a butt tuck, I need to see it." So again, I dropped my pants a little lower and turned around. My husband was looking at my furry, lower lady parts and the doctor was poking my dimpled butt. "Okay, pull'em up," he said. He told me there may be enough fat for a B cup with the flesh from the buttocks, but no one performed that type of procedure anymore. I felt like screaming at him "Then why did you look at my dimpled butt?" But I held my tongue; this office was for whispering only.

As I pulled my pants back on, he answered some of my questions about rupturing implants, implants that were known to cause cancer, and so on. He informed me of the many people in the office who have had some sort of reconstructive surgery. He seemed knowledgeable, but I was trying to gauge whether I was comfortable enough to go under the knife with him.

"Let's get you dressed and schedule another appointment," he said. "I want you to have time to talk with the woman from our business office regarding finances and insurance, and then talk to someone who has gone through this."

The second weekend after my diagnosis, my tribe was forming before my eyes. And behind it all was Adlai, who had stepped up and became a beacon of hope and laughter propelling me through each day. He was my reason to fight while the rest of my tribe kept me afloat.

When I arrived home that Friday after my appointment with the new plastic surgeon, I found a gift on the front doorstep—my friend Ann had left a couple of goodies. Ann was a Fitness Friend. The Fitness Friends were a group of 11 gals, including me, that met while exercising. When I first moved to Minnesota in 2009, I started teaching fitness classes. Ann was an active participant for several years. I confided in this group of girls a few days ago about my current situation. The decision to share was difficult. I didn't want to burden anyone, but at some point, my friends were going to find out, and I would rather it come from me. I began to think about my Fitness Friends. Their hearts were filled with love, love that ran so deeply in their souls it brought me to tears. Loyalty. Honor. Kindness. Generosity. Though it sounded cliché, each one of these women made the world a better place. They made my world a better place.

Ann left a potted sunflower and a book called Happiness. The simply illustrated book was charming and delightful. It was a reminder that Happiness could be the sound of popcorn popping, or sock skating around the house or simply the smell of freshly washed hair. I turned to the book many times during my journey, and it brought a smile to my face each time.

The following day, more goodies were waiting on my stoop. Sarah, another Fitness Friend, left a big bag of Twizzlers and a magnet. The magnet said, Dream Big. Work Hard. Be Brave. Shine Bright.

Fuck Off. Sometimes the F-bomb was the perfect word for a situation. Perhaps, at times, the F-bomb was Happiness.

Also resting on the front stoop was my first boobie box from Missouri. It was from my parents. I emptied the contents of the box onto the dining room table. Inside I found a hand-written note, a coloring book with markers, the Angel of Hope, meat sticks for Adlai and a decorative dish towel. I felt bathed in love, kindness and generosity. Despite any pity parties I would have along the way, I now had a tribe surrounding me with more love and support than I ever knew was possible. Each person in my tribe made my journey feel like they were fighting against cancer too. My journey suddenly became less lonely.

Over the weekend, Adlai and I talked several times about the plastic surgeon. The conversation went in circles.

"What do you really think about him?" I asked. "Do you think he has the experience to perform a double mastectomy with reconstructive surgery? Why did the nurse feel compelled to tell us about his extensive experience?"

Adlai always responded with, "How do you feel about him? He is going to be cutting on you not me. It doesn't matter what I think." After all the questions and discussions and brooding, I realized I didn't have the confidence in him that I wanted in a plastic surgeon. This was my life. I would forever have these fake breasts, imposters, and I didn't want them to look like a bungled mess sewn to my chest.

First thing Monday morning, I wanted more answers. Answers from someone who had been through this journey. I decided to call the breast care coordinator, and she gave me the number for the Pink Ribbon Mentors, a group of breast cancer survivors who share their experiences with newcomers. Within hours of reaching out to the Pink

Ribbon Mentors, I received a call back from one of them. We
scheduled time to talk that evening at 8 p.m.

After I hung up with the mentor, I sent my friend Katie a note.
She was also a Fitness Friend and a nurse at the clinic where I was
being treated. Her tenure at this hospital spanned more than 15 years
and she has cared for many breast cancer patients. I wanted to speak to
Katie, not only because she worked at the clinic, but I knew she would
give me an honest opinion. Katie was a sweet person who loved deeply,
but she also wasn't afraid to say Go Fuck Yourself if you needed an
attitude adjustment. Thankfully for me, she never found the need to tell
me to Go Fuck Myself. Unless I made her do burpees during a fitness
class, then she may have said it under her breath.

I asked for Katie's opinion about the medical wonderchild. She
told me he was easy on the eyes but didn't know a lot about him. She
heard that he cared a lot about his patients, but he lacked experience.
She recommended that I contact the other plastic surgeon on staff. He
had what the nurses call "Million Dollar Hands!" She also told me my
general surgeon was amazing as well. She called the two of them "The
Dream Team!"

I thanked Katie for her recommendation, and I promised
myself I would call the plastic surgeon's office Monday morning and
request to have an appointment the with the other plastic surgeon.

That evening, my Pink Ribbon Mentor talked with me for
about an hour. She had had her procedure at another clinic. She
described her surgery and chemotherapy. I was surprised to hear losing
her hair was one of the biggest obstacles for her. I couldn't care less
about my hair. If I had to go through chemo, all I cared about was not
throwing up. I wondered if that was even a possibility. Hopefully, I
wouldn't have to worry about chemotherapy. My mentor went on to
say she worked through many months of chemo treatments. My hero, I
thought to myself.

Adlai and I returned to the plastic surgeon's office. We barely sat down in the waiting room before being whisked away to one of the private rooms in back. We settled in the chairs in the doctor's office, and the nurse pelted me with most of the same questions they asked last week. I knew this time not to ask for a butt tuck especially since I remembered putting on granny panties again today. Let's face it, granny panties had become my way of life—more comfortable than the butt floss I used to wear. And I didn't care one bit. After her line of questioning, I thanked her for squeezing me in so quickly. I told her I wasn't comfortable with the other surgeon. The corners of her mouth curled in a polite smile and she said, "This is what we are here for."

After the barrage of questions, the plastic surgeon arrived. He had a thick European accent. I later found out he was Serbian. He was kind, genuine, and confident. He didn't whisper, and I felt like he wasn't hiding anything from me. I made my decision that day to go with the "Dream Team."

My new plastic surgeon walked me step by step through the procedure telling me exactly what to expect. We discussed his experience and longevity at the clinic, and he said everything was going to be fine. I felt like I was a textbook case. Snip. Snap. Snip. Snap. Done.

"I want the same size I have. I want nothing smaller, nothing bigger," I said. He literally cupped my right breast between his hands. As he jiggled my breast he said, "Don't worry. That is the easy part. I will handle it. Plus, we have a system that will give us the information we need to create the perfect size."

Then the pleasantries ended. He told me the procedure wasn't going to be easy. I appreciated his candor because the general surgeon made it sound like a simple procedure. The surgeon stood me in front of the mirror and said, "Watch. This is what's going to happen." As he explained, he sketched a football shape on my right breast with a blue highlighter. One end started at my armpit while getting wider through the middle over my nipple, and then it tapered off again at my sternum. His explanation and confidence in his job made me feel like I could manage this cancer journey despite the difficulties I was presented.

"Do you want us to try to save the nipple and reattach it?" He asked.

"No. Absolutely not," I said. In the short time that I had been diagnosed, I read a memoir about one woman who tried to have hers reattached after the surgery. She said one of her nipples fell off when she was drying off after a shower. I couldn't imagine having my nipple laying on the floor for one of my cats to bat around. "I'll wait and consider a nipple tattoo."

"Have you decided on silicone or saline implants, Nicole?"

"I don't know. I can't remember the difference. There's been so much information given to me lately; I don't have a clue," I said.

He explained that silicone implants had a more natural look and feel. He didn't need to say anything else. That answered my question. Of course I wanted something that closely resembled me. I desperately wanted something that looked and felt like the beauties that would soon be banished from my chest.

"You have one more decision to make, Nicole. We can insert the implants over the chest muscles or under the chest muscles. For active people, we recommend under the muscle to help secure them," he said.

I must have given him my best deer in headlights look because he began to explain.

"High impact aerobic activity can cause the implants to turn the wrong direction especially if the activity is done too soon after the surgery. We call this implant displacement. If we secure them under the chest muscle, you don't have to worry about displacement," he explained.

For someone as active as me, this decision was easy. I answered confidently, "Put them under the muscle."

As Adlai and I walked from the plastic surgeon's office to the general surgeon's office, I felt prepared for the battle ahead. I was ready to talk about setting up the surgery. We sat on the cheap vinyl love seat in the doctor's office not knowing the general surgeon would drop the second bomb: chemotherapy.

Boom. Bile welled deep in my gut and crawled into my throat. I swallowed hard. I hate to throw up which made the thought of chemo that much worse. I was confused. I thought my choices were lumpectomy with radiation or double mastectomy with reconstruction. He never mentioned the chemo word until today. He looked at me like I was ignorant and naïve. Apparently, I was. Because I wasn't a medical professional, I had no idea what type of cancer constituted chemo and what type of cancer didn't.

For non-medical professionals, this was what I learned about chemotherapy from my surgeon:

- If you have multiple tumors, you are a candidate for chemo
- If you have a tumor larger than 1 cm, you are a candidate for chemo
- If your lymph nodes are affected, you are a candidate for chemo

I am not a medical professional; these are not recommendations. This is just what I was told.

Nicole L. Czarnomski

He left abruptly after the shrapnel from his chemo bomb embedded into my skin. I was fighting back tears when the nurse came in 10 minutes later. I was trying to turn it into anger instead of fear. I hated crying in front of people. I associated shame with crying. I needed to get over the shame; I had cancer, not strep throat. Crying was acceptable.

The nurse reviewed a brochure with the date for surgery and the requirements prior to surgery. As she spoke, I wondered if it would be easier to stay in a bubble the night before surgery, given all the rules. I bit my tongue and didn't ask for the bubble rental though I thought it sounded appropriate. Apparently, washing with Dial or an antibacterial soap was a requirement the night before and the morning of the surgery. Gross. My skin was going to be itchy and dry. She spelled out the routine:

- Wash the surgical area with a clean washcloth the evening before and the morning of surgery. Remember to use a clean cloth each time.
- Dry yourself after the shower with a clean towel each time. Do not use the same towel.
- Wear clean pajamas the night of your surgery.

As she went through all of this, I told her my cat sleeps with me every night and has for a decade. She curls up on my chest with her little motor running. I loved this nightly ritual, but the nurse did not. The antibacterial bubble I had to create before surgery wasn't feline approved.

That was the last straw. The thought of my precious cat, my fur kid, Miss B, sleeping without me put me over the edge. The tears poured from my eyes. The nurse quickly grabbed a box of tissues and set them in front of me.

She wanted to know if I wanted to talk to the doctor about anything–essentially, she wanted to pawn off the crybaby sitting beside her. Oh, who am I kidding, I'd probably want to pawn off the girl crying hysterically too. I responded by shaking my head no and asked to leave the office. She rushed through the rest of the information. At this point, I was not processing anything. I was freaking out. The only thought bouncing around in my head right now was CHEMO.

Soon we were released from the office. Adlai and I got in the car and went home. I tried to stop crying, but I hurt deep inside my heart and my brain. The chemo news seemed just as bad as the cancer diagnosis.

I called my mother who was with my grandmother at the time. My grandma lived at an assisted living community where pets came as visitors but were not allowed to live with residents. My mom and dad took over care for Missy, my grandma's little yappy dog, when she went to assisted living. Mom took Missy to visit my grandma each week. I told my mom about the chemo and she tried to be positive, telling me all would be well. I knew she was being strong because she didn't want to upset my grandma, nor did she want to show any weakness for me.

My mom asked if I wanted to talk to grandma. I begrudgingly agreed. My mom passed the phone to my grandma who started to cry when I said hello. Grandma told me her dog no longer loved her. I heard a shuffling on the other end of the phone. My mom was back on the line. "I'm so sorry," she said. "I thought she would be happy to hear from you. Are you okay?"

"Yes," I said. And strangely, I was. My grandma was upset about her dog not loving her. We all have challenges ahead of us each day. Some of us have small hurdles and some of us have larger hurdles, but we all figure it out. We dig deep inside of our hearts and minds and we jump over those hurdles.

I made veggie burgers and French fries for dinner. I picked at the food and took tiny little bites like a little rabbit nibbling on a carrot. The lump in my throat made it hard to swallow, so I pushed the plate aside and went over to the sofa. I sat on the overstuffed, ultra-suede sofa we had owned for at least six years. It was our first major furniture purchase. It was comforting to be home on a familiar sofa. I sat slumped over with red, puffy eyes and waited for the second Pink Ribbon Mentor to call me.

At 8 p.m. sharp I received a call from her. She too gave me an hour of her time. Although the topic was depressing, she was a delight to talk to. I felt comforted to know she survived the brutal journey. We discussed chemo. She said she suffered from the fatigue, but didn't get physically ill, mostly nauseous. She too struggled with hair loss. "When my hair started falling out in chunks, I went and selected the perfect wig, and made an appointment with my hair stylist who buzzed my hair." She did say the one benefit to a wig was that it was easy to get ready in the morning. Always a silver lining. Then she asked about my surgery and was interested in why they weren't doing the chemo first. She urged me to ask more questions.

First thing Friday morning, I called my general surgeon's office. I posed the chemo/surgery surgery/chemo question. His nurse said he was in surgery, and she would have him call me post-op.

At noon, he called and said, "We should biopsy the lymph node to determine if the chemo should come first or second." I was confused. I was simply asking about the order of this procedure and why he chose the order of going into surgery first over chemotherapy. Now he was suggesting another biopsy even though I had already been to the radiologist twice. At this point, I was told the lymph node was not biopsied the first time around. They missed the node and tested fatty tissue instead.

35

When I told my general surgeon that I was confused about the situation, he told me to get a second opinion. His tone was harsh and abrasive. A second opinion. My strength was waning, and I felt like he was trying to pawn me off. It's like I was just another breast cancer case and another one would be coming down the pipeline today or tomorrow. His paycheck was already signed, so why should he care about me?

I hesitated but agreed. The general surgeon said he would initiate another biopsy at another clinic. I was at work while all of this was unfolding. By the time the other clinic called me, it was around 4:30 p.m. on Friday July 21. I was away from my desk when the call came in, and I didn't get the message until 4:45 p.m. I called back to schedule the biopsy with the alternate clinic. They asked what type of cancer I had. "I don't know, breast cancer. Isn't that in the orders the general surgeon sent over?" I asked.

"No," she said, "we need the type of cancer you have prior to scheduling the biopsy."

I hung up with her and called my general surgeon's office. The receptionist put me on hold. I listened to the generic elevator music and was getting impatient. Time was ticking, and it was Friday. I was about to spend another weekend waiting for answers. When the nurse interrupted the elevator music, I learned I had invasive ductal carcinoma, Nottingham grade 2. The clinic hadn't determined the stage because they didn't know if the cancer had spread to my lymph nodes, though it was likely. I called the new clinic and shared this news. They asked a question that only a medical professional could understand, and I said I didn't know. "This is the only information they gave me," I said.

"Well we can't schedule an appointment unless we know this information," she replied.

She then said, "I guess you are probably really hoping to get an appointment."

"Ah, yes, please," I said with only a hint of sarcasm in case it was a recorded line.

"Okay, we'll schedule you and get the information on Monday. Make sure to follow up with us," she said. Perfect I thought. The receptionist then said, "Okay, we can't just schedule you for a biopsy though, we'll have you meet with a nurse who can then set up an appointment with a surgeon who will order the biopsy." By now, my frustration started to boil out of control.

She decided to schedule me for Thursday with the nurse. "Fine," I said. I called back to my original surgeon's office at 5:10 p.m. The receptionist reminded me it was after five and the office was closed. I asked for voicemail and she informed me voicemail was not an option.

I got off the phone and called the Breast Care Coordinator at my original general surgeon's office because she had voicemail. The message I left was manic. My words were a confusing jumble, and after I hung up the phone, I was embarrassed and pissed off. Once again it was Friday, and for the fourth weekend in a row, I was waiting for answers. This was starting to feel personal. As I drove home, I mulled over the events of the day. First, my surgeon requested another biopsy even though during my second visit to the radiologist, they determined there were no other masses that needed to be tested. Second, my surgeon couldn't explain the need to do surgery prior to chemo. And finally, he wanted to pawn me off to another clinic.

When I arrived home, I changed into comfy clothes and popped open a hard cider. I nibbled on crackers and cheese. I popped a few cashews in my mouth and finished dinner with several Twizzlers. I grabbed another hard cider and sat on the couch overcome by everything that transpired that day. I held my frustration deep inside until I laid my head on my pillow that night. I fell into a fitful sleep.

On Saturday, my dear friend Kathy and her granddaughter Izzy arrived at my house at 9 a.m. Izzy had a little tuft of blondish hair pulled back in a barrette, and she loved the meows, or cats, in my house. She handed me a brightly colored floral gift bag. Izzy was excited to go for a walk, so I put the bag aside and the three of us walked around my neighborhood.

The rage I harbored deep inside darted off my tongue and pierced the humid air surrounding us. I told Kathy about the biopsy and how they missed the lymph nodes during the biopsy and scored nothing but fatty tissue. I told her how my general surgeon treated me on the phone when I simply asked a question about which procedure came first, surgery or chemo. And finally, I got to talk about chemo. Kathy listened to my frustrations and tried to console me, but there was nothing she could say to take away the cancer and what the next several months were going to bring, though I was grateful to have her by my side.

At the end of the walk, she said she and two other Fitness Friends wanted to schedule meal delivery. They knew I would not be up for cooking, and they didn't know how else to help. Tears stung my eyes and kissed my eyelashes before running down my cheeks. Sometimes I cried for the shitty situation I found myself in, and sometimes I cried because of the kindness and generosity of the people around me. I wanted to be strong and not ask for help, but I knew meal delivery was going to be a blessing. They also offered to have someone come and clean my house, something I've wanted for years but felt it was overindulgent and unnecessary.

After our walk, I sought out nourishment for my ever-shrinking appetite. I choked down a fruit smoothie and half a waffle. Breakfast was usually a welcome treat each morning but shoving food into my gullet had become more and more taxing as the days passed.

When I finished breakfast, I drove to Target and shopped for my weekly groceries. I found myself staring off into nothing, missing the necessities for the week. I drove the 25 miles home in a daze, and I waited in limbo dreading the upcoming week.

After I arrived home and put my groceries away, I sat and waited, for what, I don't know. Time passed so slowly it felt like the hands on the clock were moving through molasses. I gazed at the gift bag sitting on the table, the one Izzy had given me earlier in the day. I had been stuck inside my head for hours and forgotten about the sweet gesture. I reached my hand in the bag and rifled through the tissue paper. I pulled out a beautiful silver bracelet. It had a small charm attached. It was a moon and a star engraved with the phrase, I love you to the moon and back. A flood of emotions overcame my body, paralyzing me for a few moments before my thoughts began to flow again. How did I attract this supportive and generous person in my life? This tribe of mine, gathering around me like worker bees protecting the queen, how did I get so lucky?

For years, I sabotaged relationships with friends and lovers, never feeling I was good enough for their love or adoration. I was hypercritical of myself. I ran away from problems, hoping new friends, new lovers, new jobs, new places to live would be better, easier to manage, only to discover these changes didn't make me into the person that everyone loved. This love and adoration always seemed just out of my reach. With each new home and job and relationship, I still felt inadequate. I wasn't smart enough, or pretty enough, or skinny enough. I didn't have enough money. I didn't have the right job or car or clothing. And now, at the age of 42, I had a tribe gathering around me to help me through one of life's most difficult challenges, but why? What had I done to deserve them?

First thing Monday morning, I called and left yet another message with the breast care coordinator. She had been out on vacation last week, so it took her until mid-afternoon to return my call. She apologized for the delay but wanted to do some investigating before she could explain what had happened.

When I heard her voice, I was relieved. She said she was very sorry to have caused confusion, and they had made a mistake. "The radiologist who performed your first biopsy was on vacation when you were in for the second ultrasound. When the alternate radiologist didn't see anything suspicious the second time, he didn't believe there should be another biopsy," she said. Her tone was genuine as she apologized for the mistake. She spoke to me like I was her sister. I felt better about the situation and regained trust in the Dream Team. They had an opening available for me the following morning for biopsy number two.

That night, Adlai and I sat at the dining room table and wrote out several questions. I was going to grill the surgeon about the process they were recommending. I knew this was imperative for me to continue trusting him and his recommendations.

Tuesday morning, Adlai and I went to the appointment together. We waited in his office for only a few minutes. When he arrived, he cracked a joke and gave me a smile. It was the first time I had ever seen a smile on his face. He answered most of my questions but stopped me when I started asking about radiation and chemo affecting the implants post-surgery. Very gently he said, "Nicole, we need to focus on the two tumors. We'll worry about the rest later. The tumors are the most important thing. You are young and strong, and you are going to recover quickly from all of this." He said in six months I would look back on all of this and it would simply be a memory.

I interrupted him. This was important to me. I wanted to know about chemo and radiation, and I felt he should answer my questions. I asked about nausea and getting sick from chemo. He said, "Yes, some people do suffer from vomiting." I interrupted him again, and said I was going to need something for nausea. He reassured me that I would be fine, and that I would endure about two to three months of chemo. He was genuine and patient when speaking to me. Slowly my tense nerves began to relax.

After my meeting with the surgeon, I was prepped for the ultrasound and second biopsy. The radiologist came in, sat down and looked me in the eyes. "The last time you were in, we were really focused on those two tumors," he said. "Today, we are going to biopsy that lymph node, and we hope it's going to come back negative. But if it doesn't, we're going to get you through this."

That evening I went for a walk. I used that time alone to visualize cancer leaving my body. I walked for over an hour. I pumped my arms back and forth hoping each stride would release little bits of the tumor. The walk was like meditation, and I chose to continue walking all throughout my journey even through some of the darkest days of chemotherapy.

After my walk, I took off my shirt and noticed the tape they used to cover the biopsy site rubbed the skin tissue raw again, only this time it was much worse. I had large red welts from the bandage. One of the welts was bleeding, so I peeled off the bandage, cringing when sweat trickled over the raw skin. As I inspected the skin, I contemplated the second opinion with clinic number two. I had kept my appointment scheduled even though I felt better about the care I was receiving at the first clinic.

I received a phone call from the second clinic the following day. "Good morning. Is this Nicole?" the woman on the phone asked.

"Yes," I said.

"This is Kayla, and we scheduled your appointment for tomorrow incorrectly, so I need to reschedule your appointment."

I didn't understand what was wrong with the appointment. "How did you schedule it incorrectly?" I asked.

"It needs to be scheduled differently on a new calendar," she said.

"A different calendar?" I asked irritation flooding my voice.

"Yes, you'll still be at the breast clinic, but on a different calendar," Kayla said. She went on and on about the specific calendars they use for their providers and getting this appointment scheduled correctly. I sat on the other end of the phone rolling my eyes and sighing every few seconds. If she noticed, she had a stellar way of ignoring or hiding it. I let her reschedule the appointment.

She asked if I could speak to a nurse today. The nurse had several questions to ask and the phone call would take about 30 minutes. I said yes, even more annoyed. I had already missed a lot of work because of all the appointments and phone calls, and I was struggling to keep up with daily tasks. I tried to remind myself that work had to take a spot on the back burner because my body was preparing to battle cancer and my life needed to come first.

During my call with the nurse, she asked about my medical history, my medications, past surgeries and family history. "You'll need to have your regular physician and your general surgeon release your records," she said.

To release records, both clinics needed my signature. This was going to require me traveling to two different clinics in two different towns and have the records sent by Friday, which was now only two days away.

That Friday, I was scheduled for a two-hour appointment with another nurse at the new clinic to discuss their recommendations for breast cancer treatment. I was exhausted from all the appointments, phone calls, and running around, so the following day, I cancelled my appointment with the new clinic and continued to trust in the first clinic.

While waiting for the biopsy results, living a "normal" life was difficult. Finding my exercise groove was a challenge, exhaustion seemed to take over. Concentrating on tasks at work was also challenging. My day to day life was a constant reminder of failure, as if this disease was my fault. I took birth control pills for too many years. I didn't eat the right food. I criticized my body. Accepting the cancer diagnosis made me feel like I had done something wrong. If I would have chosen a different path years ago, would I still be in this predicament?

The phone call came at 3 p.m. on a Friday. It was good news for a change; the first good news in four weeks. There were no traces of cancer found in the lymph node they biopsied. I exhaled like I had been holding my breath for days. A smiled appeared as I hung up the phone.

Although the doctors gave me good news Friday, it was difficult to imagine what the next several months were going to be like. I struggled to keep my thoughts in the present. I thought about having surgery and wondered about the level of pain after a double mastectomy and reconstructive surgery. Chemotherapy, another unknown, scared me. Images of me laying on the bathroom floor heaving into the toilet entered my brain more often than I wanted.

I woke up on Saturday and needed to clear the negative thoughts in my mind. Instead of running, I went for a walk. I left my earbuds and music at home, allowing me to be alone with my thoughts. This walk was instrumental in changing my thought patterns. Somewhere along the way, I let go of feeling at fault and feeling sorry for myself and started looking for the things that were important. A healthy body was important, so eating well, exercising, and keeping a healthy mind set were paramount. Criticizing my plump and dimpled rump, my short legs, my saggy boobs and my squishy tummy wasn't healthy. Instead of criticizing her, I needed to love her because it was a vessel housing my soul. I needed to spend more time nurturing her.

A part of my body was about to be banished forever. Boobs the plastic surgeon said were perfectly symmetrical—gone. Boobs with true nipples to be titillated during sex—gone. Boobs that at one time won a wet t-shirt contest during spring break at South Padre Island—gone.

I can't recall now if it was my freshman or sophomore year in college when my ladies won the prize. Me and three other gals from college made the 18-hour road trip in my friend's maroon Crown Victoria. Each day of the trip, we drank ourselves silly. The only reason I can remember anything from the trip was because I had photos to prove it. Photos of us all drinking green beer for St. Patrick's Day, chugging wine from a bottle, and smoking cigarettes like we were all addicted. Thankfully, I have zero photos from the wet t-shirt contest. (I hope no photos of me exist from that contest.) And thankfully, cell phones were rare and social media was non-existent. Though now, a shameful thing to admit, me standing on stage being sprayed with a hose like some twenty-dollar hooker, it seemed horrifying to let these award winning and delicate beauties become waste. Burned in an incinerator. I wanted to hold on tight and tell the girls how sorry I was for treating them so poorly. Criticizing them. It didn't matter. They didn't care. Soon, two silicone imposters would take their place.

Not only did my self-image need a boost, but so did my marriage. It wasn't that my marriage was bad; I was in love with my husband. It just wasn't a priority. Writing projects took over my life, leaving my husband to find activities and other friends to keep him busy. On this walk, I realized, if I wanted him by my side, I would need to show him how important he was to me.

Valuable lessons were being learned with each passing day.

The Friday before my surgery I had to meet with a nurse practitioner who could deem me ready to go under the knife. It seemed odd to meet with another person who was not part of my surgical care team. I had never met this nurse practitioner before in my life, yet she was my ticket to the party. Why couldn't the surgeon decide if I was ready to be sliced and diced? I wondered if this woman held a special key to my journey.

The nurse practitioner arrived with a smile and a firm handshake. She sat down and said, "It looks like you are having a double mastectomy." She said it like I chose this option because of vanity. Frustration loomed over me like a thick fog. Did she think this was an elective surgery?

I snapped at her. "My general surgeon ordered this appointment. I have breast cancer."

Tension, anxiety and anger pierced the air as the words rolled off my tongue. She told me to let the anger out. "It's okay to be angry; let it go and move on." This was infuriating. I had cancer. Who was she to act like a therapist? I was allowed to be angry.

She asked who my regular physician was and why I wasn't visiting with her for this pre-op appointment. I explained how my general physician told me the lump I found was nothing. "My doctor called my lump 'smooth and non-worrisome'," I said disgusted. I went on to tell her how my physician told me the American Cancer Society recommended getting your first mammogram at age 45 if there was no history of breast cancer in your family. "I took her advice!" I exclaimed. "And now I have cancer and probably have had it for at least a couple of years!"

Her voice was soft and hushed when she told me to let it out, all of it, so it wouldn't ruin my life. This wasn't therapy! The nerve of this woman.

"I am a breast cancer survivor too, and I've had it three times," she said. I immediately let my guard down and felt an instant connection to her. She did hold a special key to my journey. She knew what I was feeling three times over.

She praised me for choosing a double mastectomy. It wasn't that I needed the praise, because whatever she said wasn't going to change my mind, but it was comforting to hear I was making a good decision from a breast cancer survivor. She continued the exam by asking the same questions every other health care provider had asked in the last couple of weeks. These questions were getting old.

Nicole L. Czarnomski

I left her office after the barrage of questioning and had the weekend to daydream about the upcoming surgery. I had three days left before my body would change forever, part of me erased and never to return.

The Sunday before my surgery, the Fitness Friends and I gathered at Brewski's, a bar owned by Marcia, one of the Fitness Friends. It was one last Hoo-Rah before my surgery on Wednesday. I thought we were gathering for a drink, a bite to eat, and some girl time. Instead I had a big surprise waiting for me.

We were gathered around a large round table talking and drinking. Without a clue as to what was happening behind me, Sarah hoisted a gigantic basket, and set it in front of me. It was overflowing with pre-op and post-op goodies along with remedies to help me during chemo. I dug through the basket to find soft, button-down jammies and button-down shirts along with soft and cozy head scarves for when I lose my hair. There was lotion, books, silly cat butt magnets, a darling little hat, artwork with a positive affirmation, wine, socks and so many other goodies.

The lump in my throat started to grow, and I wondered how I would ever eat the salad I had ordered. We laughed and conversed and suddenly I realized my mind had stopped sprinting down the rabbit hole. I was laughing and giggling like all was well in good in the world. Cancer had nothing on me and my tribe!

Monday evening, my parents arrived. They had a long, boring drive from Missouri, through Iowa, and they were ready to help me

47

through the first leg of my journey. My next pre-op appointment was scheduled for Tuesday, August 8, which was also my last day at work for the next three months. It was the sentinel node scan, another scan to test lymph nodes for cancer. The sentinel nodes were the first few nodes where tumors drained. The radiologist had to inject radioactive liquid into my nipple that funneled into my lymphatic system. The radioactive fluid helped highlight cancer in the imaging following the injection.

My parents took me to the appointment. We arrived at a doctor's office in the middle of a residential area. It wasn't memorable from the outside, but when I walked into the building, the walls were adorned with brightly colored abstract paintings. I checked in and took a seat so I could get lost in the beauty of the artwork. I was summoned for the procedure before I had time to surrender to the artwork and fully absorb each painting.

First, I had photos taken of my breasts, and then the radiologist forewarned me of the procedure. I was having a sentinel node scan to detect cancer in the lymph nodes. He warned me about the painful procedure. "The pain will be brief, but intense," he said softly. I blew off the warning. I had a high tolerance for pain.

"Why must you do the sentinel node scan if there was no cancer found in the lymph nodes when I had the second biopsy?" I asked.

He took both my hands and gently squeezed them. "Nicole, you can't go down this path. This is a procedure doctors do to everyone with breast cancer. This procedure is not unique to you. Everyone in the country does this," he said. My trust in him waivered as he stammered through the explanation.

He urged me to trust him and stop asking questions. I wondered if I was one of those patients that doctors joked about—was I

Nicole L. Czarnomski

the problem child? The bully? Maybe he needed to work on his confidence. I accepted his excuse with much trepidation and lay down on the machine prepared for the painful procedure. He apologized again and began to describe the procedure. "You'll feel a poke and sting and a lingering burning sensation," he said as his brows furrowed.

This was a complete and total under exaggeration. The procedure felt like someone filled a syringe with molten hot lava from a volcano and held the needle over a blue flame until it started to glow. The needle was then inserted into my nipple in four separate places. He referred to my nipple as having numbers on the clock. The blazing hot needle was inserted at 12:00, 3:00, 6:00 and 9:00. The pain was so severe I began to grind my teeth as tears surfaced at the edge of my eyelids. The nipple scalding procedure took about 60 seconds, maybe 90 seconds. If it would have lasted any longer, I would have passed out from the pain. True story.

This was followed by almost two hours of imaging completed in a giant machine that looked like an MRI machine. The images showed where the lymph nodes were located which was crucial for my surgery the following day. When all the tests were completed, I had been cleared for surgery. I had a few hours to go home, shower with anti-bacterial soap to create the perfect bubble around my body and stay clear of any felines.

Nicole L. Czarnomski

# Part 2: Bilateral Mastectomy with Reconstruction

# Bye Bye Boobies

August 9, 2017. I was surprisingly calm as my husband drove my parents and me to the hospital at 7 a.m. It was time to say goodbye to my breasts.

I checked-in at the front desk and waited to be called for phase one. I started to fidget while I waited. "Nicole," the nurse said looking in my direction. I looked up at her.

"Yes, that's me," I said. My spine straightened as if there were a metal rod holding up each vertebra. I felt a surge of heat cross my face and then my whole body turned cold and goose bumps erupted on my skin as I walked into the room.

I was instructed to undress and put on a purple, paper-like gown. While I waited for my surgeon, the ice-like feeling in my veins melted, and I realized the blueprints, the upcoming drugs, the cutting, the removing, and the rebuilding were all good things. A second chance on life. The two doctors in charge of my fate were about to perform a procedure they could probably do in their sleep, though I hoped they wouldn't, and by the end of the day I would be cancer free.

Moments later, my plastic surgeon arrived and greeted me. He had a small plastic tackle box that looked like the tackle box I used in art school. When he opened it, there was a rainbow hiding inside. He had an array of permanent Sharpie markers. There were as many colors as Hobby Lobby had on the shelf. "Pick a color," he said in his thick Serbian accent.

"Oh, orange," I responded, "That's my favorite color!" He smiled and quickly plotted the course along both breasts. He drew a football shape starting close to the armpit and ending close to my sternum. My nerves tightened when I realized there was a lot of skin tissue about to become trash.

He smiled and gathered his art box. "I have another surgery this morning, but I will be back late morning to check on you. Go ahead and get dressed. The nurse will be right with you," he said. He left for his first surgery.

Pre-op lab work was next on the docket. My parents and my husband, my entourage, returned to the main floor. It was a peculiar feeling walking the halls of the clinic before many of the staff members and patients had arrived. I felt like I was Hans Solo leading the troops through the long halls of the Death Star minus the dramatic music. We were preparing for battle. Yes, we. We were all in it together just like mom and Adlai said weeks ago when I was diagnosed. After checking in, we sat quietly in the waiting room, no one knowing what to say to me.

As we waited in the waiting room to have labs completed, I was concerned there would be no pee to give for the lab work. I wasn't allowed to drink or eat past midnight the night before, and earlier that morning I had to pee so bad my bladder ached. The stream of urine that morning kept coming like there were back up bladders holding more urine than normal. I had cotton mouth and wondered if my bladder was feeling the drought as well.

A woman who looked unhappy with life walked out and called my name. I hoped she wouldn't take it out on me. She looked at me with a straight face and handed me the pee cup. "Please put this in the red bin when you are finished," she said. I wondered how many urine and blood samples she had to deal with daily. Maybe I would be mad at the world too if I managed pee cups and bloody needles day in and day out.

I situated myself over the toilet with the small plastic cup. It was the size of a Dixie cup. I don't know why they can't provide a wider cup for women. Why should our stream be expected to hit such a small cup? Just when I thought there may not be any urine to spare, a blast sprayed into the cup. I tried to suppress the stream, but I peed all over my hand. Thankfully, some landed in the cup. I put the cup in the bin and nearly scrubbed the skin off my hands remembering I was supposed to be in a bubble until surgery.

The pee test was to see if I was pregnant. I found this amusing and terrifying. I was having my period at the time and had taken two pregnancy tests already. Yes, I panicked about a week prior to surgery because I hadn't gotten my period. I was forced to stop taking the pill when I was diagnosed, so my system was off. And, yes, despite the cancer, I was still having sex with my husband, so I was terrified at the thought of pregnancy. First, this would postpone cancer treatment, and second, a little bundle of joy right now did not sound very joyful to me. My husband and I chose to live our lives childless, and we wanted it to remain that way. After the urine test, the technician also drew a vial of blood, and I was dismissed from part two of my pre-op appointments.

My entourage and I were instructed to go to another wing of the hospital for the needle localization with the radiologist. Needle was never a fun word for me, so I was anxious going into this appointment. The radiologist was also the most hated doctor on my team at this point. He missed the lymph node during the first biopsy, then he performed the sentinel node scan which was beyond painful, and now, the needle localization.

For non-medical professionals, this is what I learned from my radiologist. A needle-localized biopsy is a procedure using thin guide wires to mark the location of a tumor so it can be surgically cut out in surgery. The doctor uses an ultrasound probe to place the wire in or around the affected area. After the wires are in place, a mammogram is completed.

This procedure started with the ultrasound. The radiologist probed around the far-right area of my right breast and into my armpit. The closer they were to my armpit the more anxious I became. My palms started sweating as I imagined needles poking out of my breast while being smashed during a mammogram. The ultrasound technician and the doctor started whispering again. By this point, I knew whispering wasn't good.

I stared up at the artwork on the ceiling. Those same trees, streams, color blocking, butterflies and other photos adorned the ceiling that I had seen twice before during the biopsies. I tried to focus on the beauty of the artwork until the needles started going into my armpit.

The pain didn't measure up to the sentinel node scan, but my body felt assaulted. There was pulling and probing and pushing and skin pricks. I focused on my breathing. Smell the roses. Blow out the candle. Repeat. It took about 40 minutes to mark both tumors. Thin wires stuck out from my armpit like elongated acupuncture needles. When the needles were in place, I was walked down the hall to receive a mammogram, where I would become a contortionist.

The radiologist led me to a room with the dark-haired young woman who would perform the mammogram. I remember my grandma saying many years ago, "Mammograms are like putting your tits in a ringer." She was right. They were uncomfortable but with needles protruding from my skin, I felt like this was hitting below the belt. I had breast images taken while I stood cocking my chest to the side and leaning as far forward as possible so the camera could take a picture of the armpit. The tech took multiple photos each time telling me, "not quite."

I struggled to suppress tears, to be strong. I was hurting, my body contorted into positions it wasn't made to be in. I was a skewered gummy bear.

When I returned to the waiting room, I couldn't look at my family. I was ragged, in pain and stressed. I fought back tears as I chomped the side of my lip. Not even an F-bomb could express the sheer terror I was experiencing. The silent cancer tumors were pushing closer to the finish line, I was dragging myself inch by inch to catch the disease, to fight and overcome its nastiness. Would I survive this God-awful journey?

We returned to another waiting room sitting in silence. My pre-op room was being prepared for me. When the nurse finally called my name, I stood up and slogged over. My legs were heavy, each step felt like I was stepping into quicksand. I approached my pre-op room and cloaked myself in another stiff, purple gown. I longed for pre-op drugs, desperate to fall asleep. I no longer wanted to be conscious of anything around me.

Shortly after I undressed for surgery, a soft-spoken anesthesiologist with a southern drawl entered my room and began asking me questions about my medical history, all of which I had answered before. It should have comforted me knowing each doctor wanted to hear my history to make sure he or she didn't miss anything, but I was annoyed or maybe scared as my mind see-sawed back and forth from fear to strength. Each doctor visiting me meant I was one step closer to surgery. I answered politely as the anesthesiologist continued her line of questions. She told me there were two anesthesiologists on duty, and they would be duking it out in the parking lot to see which doctor would be giving me my pre-op cocktail. Duking it out in the parking lot? She must have known I needed to laugh. I told her three times in the five minutes that I didn't want to throw up.

"I will be very angry if I throw up! I will hunt you down if I so much as a dry heave. What can you give me for nausea?" I asked.

In her sweet southern drawl, she said, "I'll do everything I can to keep you from being ill, but I can't promise anything." She excused herself and said someone would be with me shortly with my medications.

I was given an IV on the top of my hand. They started me with saline, and finally, liquid luck. It was medication to help me relax. While I waited, my entourage was invited to my room. The four of us chatted about nothing, just words to help keep my mind from thinking about the upcoming procedure.

Enter: The Dream Team. My general surgeon, plastic surgeon, and radiologist stood by my bedside while my entourage stood at the foot of my bed. The room felt like it was closing in on me. Even with the liquid luck, I felt like a caged animal. The doctors were ready to have a look at the blueprints and the wires dangling from my upper right breast and armpit. My family all looked at me wide-eyed.

"Um, 'scuse me. A little privacy," I said. My family stepped out, so I could bare my chest in front of three men who had been strangers just weeks ago. It was an odd feeling. I kicked out my family, my flesh and blood, my husband who had seen me naked for years, but I was allowing three strange men to gawk at my skewered fun bags. Oh, what a world.

They were all impressed with the circuit board that was now tucked in my right breast and armpit. They discussed the blueprints drawn in orange marker. Afterward, they covered my ladies and my family was invited back to my room. My general surgeon said they would start surgery within the hour. Thank God. It was finally happening. The Dream Team was going to help catapult me to the finish line and blow past the disease that had gotten a jump start on the race.

A different anesthesiologist came in and introduced herself. I had no idea what her name was. Her accent was so thick I couldn't understand her. She must have won the fight in the parking lot. I begged her to please make sure I was given anti-nausea medication. She added the cocktail to the bag attached to my IV. Moments later, delirium. I was transported to an alternate reality.

As the team wheeled me into the operating room, bright white lights flooded my vision. Slow, deliberate blinking eyelids. I could no longer keep them open. The lights dimmed, and I drifted off to sleep.

I've heard waking up from local anesthesia is like waking up from a coma. A thick, hazy fog shrouded my mind and kept me guessing as to if I survived surgery or plunged to my death. Slow, deliberate blinks, open, close, open, close. The room came into focus. I was in a large private hospital room at the end of a hallway. One by one, family members appeared. My mother hovered over me, and I asked her the three magic questions. *Was I alive or dead?* She responded quietly, with a smile, "You're alive." *Did they go straight to implants or did they use expanders?* (Expanders are temporary fluid sacks filled weekly so the skin can stretch slowly.) "Straight to implants." *Did they find cancer in the lymph nodes?* "Yes, I am so sorry." She softly told me the surgery lasted five hours, two more than planned. While my plastic surgeon was finishing his handiwork, the pathology report came back from the lab with devastating news. There were trace amounts of cancer found in three lymph nodes. The lab insisted on removing more lymph nodes, so they could be tested.

The thought of cancer in my lymph nodes paralyzed me, crushed my spirit. Despite my foggy brain, I was cognizant enough to wonder about lymphedema and the effects of losing lymph nodes. What did this mean for my future? The thought slowly faded like an old newspaper.

She read the disappointment in my eyes. "The doctors said not to worry, Nicole. They didn't take out many of the nodes. Your surgeon believes you will be fine and most likely won't suffer from lymphedema," she said.

My doctors must have been alerted when I woke up. They came to check on me. Both surgeons said everything went very well and that I shouldn't worry about the lymph nodes. They expected me to make a full recovery. I remembered I had brought a bag of chocolates for my care team. I offered up candy and thanked them for saving my life. They both smiled and took a piece of chocolate and ambled out of the room.

It was difficult to write about the time immediately following surgery because of the drugs, but my parents said I was in good spirits. They said I was excited to have the PPs! Pain pills and perky boobs! My mom said I wasn't in a lot of pain, but I did experience some muscle spasms which was normal.

I remembered my Fitness Friend, Katie, who stopped by my room after her shift. She was the friend who gave me the advice about the Dream Team. I was secretly sad she wasn't my nurse, but I knew she had probably just finished a long shift at the hospital and dealt with a lot of needy patients. She wasn't my nurse, but she still pulled some strings to get me a large, quiet, private room at the end of the hall. She made sure I was assigned the best nurses on duty. From what I remember, Katie was in my room for a long time talking with me and my family; Katie felt like a member of my family that day.

I sucked on ice chips and sipped water, then needed to pee every hour after all the IV fluids that had been pumped into my body. I pushed the nurse call button what seemed like a hundred times that night, and each nurse who helped me was amazing. They always had a smile. Always.

I didn't get violently ill from the multiple cocktails fed to me by the anesthesiologist, not even one dry heave. That was pure happiness. It should be added to my Happiness book.

Within hours, I graduated from ice chips and water to Jell-O and broth. The following morning, I was relaxed and happy, until I found out I was being evicted that day…by noon! I was afraid of the aftermath. I didn't want the drugs to wear off. I didn't want to know what was under my gown. I remember feeling like my boobs were larger than a size C and felt like they were almost bumping my chin.

Late morning, the nurse instructed me to walk the halls, ten, maybe twenty feet was all she asked of me. She taught my mother how to empty my drains. Hanging from my body, the drains were small, football-shaped, rubber containers to hold fluid excreted from my body.

The tubes the doctors inserted into the incision were about eight inches long. The drains had to be emptied every four hours. Once my mom felt comfortable with the crash course on drains, a nurse brought in a wheelchair for me. I told her to put the remaining candy in the nurse's station and to enjoy the chocolate when times were tough. My dad pushed the wheelchair towards the exit and my husband brought the car around. As I wrapped the seat belt around my body, I put the pink boobie pillow under the chest belt in between each mound to protect the new silicone gel imposters. I don't remember much of the drive except for when we hit potholes. Ouch! It was incredibly uncomfortable but I wanted to be home so I could begin the healing process.

The days following surgery I was like a newborn kitten mewing for food and water and playtime. My mom prepared meals to ensure my tummy was full and my dad cleaned up the dishes. I napped on the sofa in the warm sunlight that streamed through the big picture window in my living room. They became servants catering to my every need.

My body was satiated with extra-strength Tylenol for pain. I never once popped a hardcore narcotic to reduce discomfort. On a few occasions I experienced uncomfortable muscles spasms and downed a couple of muscle relaxers, but I never finished that bottle of pills either.

Exercise was critical for my recovery. Unfortunately, it wasn't the type of exercise I had been accustomed to as a high school and college athlete. It wasn't even close to what this 42-year-old was used to doing. Walking my fingers up the wall like a leggy spider multiple times per hour was critical for arm mobility, especially on the right side. I later found out that 18 lymph nodes were removed, causing axillary cording to form under my right armpit. (Cording is a ropelike structure that forms under the axilla and can extend down the arm and hand.) Finger walking sounded simple, but it was critical for healing. If I neglected to complete this task, my arms may be pinned down as if I were wearing a strait jacket. Okay, that was a slight exaggeration, but it was good motivation to keep my fingers walking all those times I didn't want to.

Prior to surgery, I would spend my evenings logging miles on my running shoes. I jogged around my town for three to five miles several times a week typically with Lady Gaga pumping through my earbuds. Now, my main form of exercise was walking, which proved to be a laborious task, so I used it to build up strength, gaining more distance with each walk.

My first walk was halfway to the end of our driveway, about ten feet. Exhausted, I sat gingerly down on a lounge chair my parents bought me, until I could manage another ten feet. It wasn't long before I made it twenty feet—to the end of the driveway. My parents cheered for me every step of the way and congratulated me like I had just finished a marathon.

When it was time for this little kitten to bathe, my mom had to help. We had purchased a shower stool, and a handheld shower head to make it easier. The first time I stripped down for a shower, I felt damaged and broken, unable to look at my chest. I desperately wanted to know if it was bungled and clumsy looking. Would I be the next guest star on the reality television show, Botched? I wanted to know just how good the doctor with million-dollar hands was, but I couldn't look at myself.

"How do I look mom?" I asked in a guarded voice. Her facial expression was genuine. "You look really good; the doctors did a great job, Nicole. You have nothing to worry about," she said.

A gentle spray of warm water speckled my breasts. My eyes were the size of saucers as I sucked air into my lungs and held my breath. "No! No! No! Stop!" I screamed.

"What! What's wrong?" she asked.

"Are you supposed to get my breasts wet?" I asked.

"It's okay. Yes, they want you to shower and keep the area clean. Relax," she said.

My body recoiled again as the water gently sprayed my chest. I lathered my body swiftly and mom helped rinse the soap off. I climbed out of the tub, and she gently toweled my whole body. After the shower, she took great care in blow drying my long, thick hair.

Day after day, I grew stronger and gained a more substantial appetite. The walks I took were short and slow, but I continued to set small goals. Past the driveway, five, 10, 15 feet and back.

I endured hairy armpits and the pesky drains, or tea bags as my father called them, that continued to fill up hour after hour.

By day four, the left drain totaled 15ml of fluid in a 24-hour period which meant it was time for the removal. The right side was steadily pumping out fluid. To have the drains removed, I had to wait until there was less than 30ml in a 24-hour period. The nurses said this process usually took five to 10 days.

Since lefty scored 15ml after day four, my parents took me to the plastic surgeon's office. She was shocked at the minimal amount that had been collected and was concerned it wasn't being emptied correctly. A tutorial was given again, and I was sent home with both drains securely fastened into my armpits.

We had the same results the following day, so I called and scheduled another appointment. On day five, the left drain was going to be evicted. When I arrived at the clinic, my nurse led me down the hall and to the doctor's office at the end. Once we were in the office, I sat in the reclining chair, gingerly shed my shirt and opened my mastectomy camisole. She instructed me to reach my left arm up and over my head; it was still stiff from surgery. I held it up like a school kid waiting to be called on in class.

She pinched the tube between her fingers and started tugging so she could see the stitches. A deep stabbing pain shot into my armpit. She tugged on the drain tube. Snip, snip, the stitches were cut. A blue flame of pain shot through my armpit. My breath quickened, sweat droplets beaded on my forehead, my mind was dizzy, unable to think or process the situation.

The nurse encouraged me to breathe as I started to hyperventilate. She tugged at the tube and pulled an eight-inch tube from inside my body. Tears gushing from my eyes like a torrential down pour, I started wailing. Her voice kind, gentle, she told me to let it out. Crying was acceptable, it was standard practice. I sobbed and sobbed with great force. Nothing could stop my chest from heaving. When I thought I may pass out from the intense pain, it was finally over.

Not one doctor or nurse mentioned drain removal being so painful. Why wasn't I given local anesthetic? In the moments immediately following the pain, I was enraged. I lowered my arm and sat up. I started laughing hysterically at the brutal pain I just endured. I laughed and laughed and told her I wasn't going to let her take out the other drain. Ever. I was going to leave it in place. I told her I didn't care how rank my armpit became, that damn drain was now a part of me, another appendage. She laughed with me and said she hadn't ever had anyone react that way. Drain removal was usually the easiest part. How could this be? I wondered if she thought I was fabricating the pain.

Both of us laughed down the hall. When, we got to the lobby, she said she would see me in a few days. "Nope," I responded. "Not coming back. Ever."

With left drain out, it was easier to extend my arm up over head when I walked my fingers along the wall. Soon I was able to reach my left arm straight up in the air again, like I had never had surgery.

The right drain did exactly what I asked when I was having lefty removed. It stayed put. It was still siphoning 40-50 ml in a 24-hour period. It was depressing. I had no idea how long the drain was going to hang out in there. A typical drain remained inside for five to 10 days following surgery. A little part of me was singing Halleluiah because I wasn't ready to experience the same pain in my right armpit, but the other part of me wanted to be finished with this phase of my journey. I knew without the drain, it would be easier to do my exercises for mobility.

My parents hung out with me each day, mom diligently emptying the right drain, making sure I was comfortable. She continued to prep meals, and dad cleaned up the mess. We were so grateful when a few of my Fitness Friends brought over meals while they were in town. Sarah whipped up a homemade chicken pot pie that was delicious. She also brought a taco salad. My friend Carrie delivered stuffed green peppers along with several cucumbers and zucchinis from her garden. My friend Katie brought tater tot hot dish. I was lucky to have all these amazing people in my life, all sharing in the healing process.

Ten days after my surgery I was getting along very well. I was walking farther, taking shorter naps, and reaching for things in the cabinets and in the refrigerator. Progress. It felt good. But this good feeling was distressing. The better I felt the less I needed my parents help which meant they would be leaving soon.

I was terrified to be alone. What if I were to get an infection? What about the right drain? She wasn't out yet. How would I empty it by myself? How would I manage my house? Cleaning. Cooking. Doing laundry. They all seemed like daunting tasks.

Prior to their departure, a deluge of emotions pulsed inside of me like a throbbing thumb after its been hit with a mallet. I wanted my parents to move from their home of 30 plus years in Missouri to Minnesota. Live in our spare bedroom. It sounded reasonable. Then, I wanted to move back to Missouri or simply fake another illness. I would have said anything to get them to stay, but I knew it was time.

There was a certain magic about my parents. My Popps cracked jokes nonstop. He found it amusing that I couldn't scrub or shave my armpits, so he teased me about having to sit up-wind from me. And my drains, he always referred to them as teabags, and he was right. They looked like little teabags hanging out from my armpits. His anecdotes brought so much laughter throughout the week. What a blessing. He was even brave enough to walk with me to the Mayo Clinic mastectomy store so I could purchase a special camisole for my new jugs.

As for my mom, it wasn't only about the chores and errands. She was comforting when I needed it most. For the first three days, I was too afraid to look at myself in the mirror before my daily shower, but she reassured me that I was still beautiful, and the doctors had done an amazing job on the reconstruction. On day three, I finally had strength and courage to look at the surgeons' handiwork. She was right. My boobs looked wonderful despite the swelling and incision from armpit to sternum. The strength and grace I had to weather this storm came from a lifetime of their love and support. This had been a devastating chapter in my life, but so much beauty had come from this one special journey.

Wednesday morning, I stood in the driveway watching as they loaded their car to prepare for the eight-hour trek home. They each gave me a big, but gentle hug. They climbed in the car, and I blew them goodbye kisses as they backed out of the driveway.

Thank you or I'm grateful are two sentiments that languish mid-air when I speak them, not quite honoring how I feel about my parents. They deserved more, but I didn't know how to say it, so I decided I would make it my mission to live my life giving to others with the same unconditional love, support, and generosity they have given me all the years.

# Drain Drama

As I recovered, days churned like a spinning wheel; I never really knew if it was Monday or Friday. My fingers crawled up walls, my legs carried me for 10, 15- and 20-minute walks. I took pride in finally being able to do my household chores. I napped with cats and prepared meals, looking forward to Adlai coming home from work each day.

By day 12, the right drain continued to pump fluid from my surgery, two days more than expected. My thoughts were filled with remorse. In my head, I apologized for telling the nurse I wanted to leave the right drain securely attached because of the excruciating pain I felt when the left one was removed. I had jinxed ole Righty.

On day 15, when the drain had 30 ml of fluid filling the container, I had had enough. The goal was to be lower than that for at least two straight days. I wholeheartedly believed Righty wanted to take up permanent residence in my armpit because Lefty scared the living shit out of her.

Righty clung to me like a rock climber ascending a vertical mass of rock. No matter what I told her, she wasn't giving me a vacate notice. I tried to bribe her with pain pills and a Valium for the removal, but she insisted on producing fluid and staying comfortably wrapped inside my chest cavity.

Research. I needed to read the forums. I searched WebMD, the perfect site for hypochondriacs, and the most hated site by medical professionals. I read about a woman who spent 19 days with her drains! Then, another woman had her drains for four weeks. I was now terrified, dangling from the rock face wondering if I was going to regain my grip. My right arm was becoming more and more difficult to raise over my head. I feared loss of mobility on the right side. I was angry at my doctors for not providing the disclaimer: when a mastectomy and reconstruction patient leaves the hospital with two drains in tow, it may take five to 10 days, or up to 20 days.

Righty, drain two, was finally removed on August 25, 16 days after my surgery. Prior to the procedure, I took a muscle relaxer, and brought Adlai with me to hold my hand. He sat next to me as I opened my camisole for the nurse. I grabbed his hand and squeezed. I winced as I lifted my right arm over my head. My arm barely lifted to my forehead. The axillary cording was thick like the roots of a tree digging deep inside the earth. The nurse, my husband and I counted down, three, two, one, snip, snip, pull! I waited for the searing pain to shoot through my chest, but I felt nothing. "All done," the nurse said.

"What?!" I exclaimed. "Done?!" Either the muscle relaxer did its job, or this drain decided to be nice to me. This called for a celebration, so my husband took me to a sushi restaurant for lunch. This was my first outing, besides doctor's appointments, since my surgery. It was divine.

Saturday, the day after my right drain was removed, I noticed the Troublemaker, aka my right breast, turned a reddish hue. I felt groggy, sluggish; an overall sense of malaise seized my body. It lasted all weekend, so Monday morning, I called my plastic surgeon for an appointment. Adlai took off work to drive me. When I opened my camisole for the doctor to inspect, he said an infection had festered up inside my Right-Hand Gal. She was seriously letting me down. (Note: it's important to refill the antibiotics given at the hospital if the drain is still present—something I neglected to do—hence the infection.)

He prescribed an antibiotic, and by Wednesday, the Troublemaker lost its reddish hue. She was still swollen, and I wondered if I had contracted Boob-a-dema, lymphedema of the breast (this swelling I later found out was known as post-surgical swelling, not Boob-a-dema.) The nurse called me that morning to check in. I told her I was feeling a little better, but my breast was swollen. She wanted me to come in again to make sure the infection was clearing up.

My Fitness Friend Tami had the day off work and chauffeured me to my appointment since I was not able to drive for six weeks post-surgery.

At the appointment, my plastic surgeon pushed and pressed and squeezed and jiggled the infected breast. When he finished his observations, he felt everything appeared normal and assured me there was no fluid buildup in the Troublemaker. I was sent home to rest until my first visit with my physical therapist.

Physical therapy was a week away. Prior to my first appointment, at the recommendation of my plastic surgeon, I called my physical therapist, a lymphedema specialist, for more information about Boob-a-dema and how to reduce swelling. She said to start wearing a compression bra, keep moving, continue walking my arms up the wall, and massage my breasts three times a day.

The compression bra was a little different from the original camisole I purchased at the mastectomy store with my dad a couple of weeks ago. Compression garments help to support the muscles and encourage them to move fluid out of the affected body part. When I returned to the mastectomy store to purchase another bra, the retail associate held up the new contraption. She gave me the choice of beige, black, or white. I picked beige. The compression bra resembled a snug, cut-off tank top like a tankini swimsuit only not cute and colorful. The opening had three bra hooks in the front. There was a zipper closure on top of the hooks that squeezed the girls in nice and tight. It was worse than Spanx. The armholes consisted of two adjustable Velcro straps about two inches wide. I knew immediately I wouldn't be getting lucky in this new undergarment.

On the phone, the physical therapist instructed me to massage both breasts above and below the incision in circular motions. The goal was to push lymphatic fluid into other lymphatic roadways and to avoid pushing lymphatic fluid to the right side of my body where the lymph nodes were short staffed. Three times a day, I took the pads of my pointer finger, middle finger and ring finger and made circular motions. Wax on, wax off, I chanted as I rubbed, hoping Boob-a-dema would not afflict my breast for much longer.

I grew tired of waxing on and off within the first two days and empathized with Daniel-son doing tedious chores at Mr. Miyagi's home. What were these massages doing for me? I was not going to become a prize karate fighter. The progress was slow, and I counted the days until I was able to have my first appointment with the lymphedema specialist.

The weekend before the next phase of my journey, my brother T.J. and his girlfriend, Angie, drove from Missouri to visit Adlai and me. The timing was perfect. I was on the mend and gaining more energy. Neither one of them had been in my neck of the woods before, so they were easily entertained.

My brother expressed an interest in visiting Slippery's Bar and Grill, located on the Mississippi River in Wabasha. The movie "Grumpy Old Men" was filmed there back in the early nineties, so it's kind of a big deal for the town. I learned that weekend that my brother loved that movie, so Adlai and I took them out to lunch.

After lunch, we took a stroll along the river and had a few Kodak moments for Facebook. I was excited to show my friends and family I was no longer a shut-in recovering from surgery. I was a free woman unencumbered by drains, aches, pains and all the unpleasant things that went along with a bilateral mastectomy and reconstructive surgery.

I savored each minute that day for many reasons. I moved to Minnesota in 2009 and this was the first time my brother had been able to come and visit me, so I wanted to enjoy his company. Plus, Angie was one of the sweetest, most kind people on earth. When I was first diagnosed, she told my mom she was going to be her rock through this journey, and she did not disappoint. She lovingly sent healing quotes via text to mom and me, and she served as a sounding board for my mother.

I was also feeling more energetic. I was healing from surgery, but chemo was just around the corner, and I had a sneaking suspicion it was going to be a brutal trek. I was trying to enjoy each moment in time as it ticked away.

# Physical Therapy

Excitement pulsed through my body during the days leading up to my physical therapy appointment. I loved the idea of healing and what this new person along my journey was going to bring me. Physical therapy was another step in my recovery, and I was ready to engage in an all-out war with cancer.

When I arrived at my appointment, I checked in with a smile pasted across my face. I couldn't wait for new information to help fix the Troublemaker. My therapist greeted me with a warm smile and led me to a small private room. We discussed the swelling, discomfort, and arm mobility. To me, healing was like getting through a tough workout. The grit and determination arrived at some point through the workout, and you fought your way through it repeating the mantra You are Stronger than You Think.

I was prepared to hit the gym and start stretching and contorting my arm to loosen the rope-like cording in my armpit. After her line of questioning, we didn't leave that small, private room. She wanted me to undress from the waist up, lie face up on the mechanical bed exposing the imposters now sewn to my chest. Hmph, I thought, maybe she had to see the destruction underneath my shirt before she could determine the best path.

I shimmied out of the compression bra and stretched out on the adjustable bed. She elevated the bed and started talking about massage techniques. She was giving me techniques to do at home to help move the lymphatic fluid. These were in addition to the wax on, wax off exercises she gave me last week on the phone.

The first massage was the strangulation method. Just kidding, kind of. The technique required me to crisscross my hands across my neck, press straight back and swoop them to the front and lift it off my clavicle. As she pressed against my neck, it was gentle and relaxing, but when I did it, I wanted to choke. This would take some practice.

The other technique was similar information to what she explained to me over the phone last week. Starting on the left breast, I was instructed to make C-shaped motion from the sternum to the left armpit. First it was the upper half, then the lower half, again fumbling around like the Karate Kid learning to wax on, wax off.

The other side, the Troublemaker, would be a little different. I needed to start at the right armpit, massage my breast all the way across my breast and sternum to the left armpit. As she was demonstrating she said, "Lymph nodes are worker bees, and since lymph nodes were removed from the right side, they are compromised and unable to move the fluid efficiently."

"There is fluid buildup?" I asked.

"Yes, but it's a special protein-based molecule that forms with water to create liquid. It's not the same fluid you are thinking of that goes into the post-surgical drains. Your left side is going to help out the right side while the right lymph nodes are still in shock." She informed me that the lymphatic system was large and would help fight lymphedema. I needed to be patient and let the wounds heal. Currently, the right lymph nodes were traumatized, so massage would assist the lymphatic system while the wounds heal.

My physical therapist spent over an hour teaching me the most effective massage techniques. There were five massages to be completed daily. She also recommended physical therapy twice a week. She said, "You are more than welcome to do them with me or with another one of our specialists." I countered quickly, "Uh, I'd like for you to do it. My plastic surgeon told me he would not allow anyone to touch me besides you."

She laughed, "That's because I am old and seasoned."

I said, "No, it makes you wise and good at what you do." I loved humble people.

After my session, she recommended a special padding with sewn in channels to go inside the bra. This would help with the flow of fluid as well. This could be purchased at the mastectomy store. She said she would have my plastic surgeon call in a prescription for it.

That night, I wanted to review my massages with Adlai, and I told him it would be helpful if he could assist me. My physical therapist had also sent me home with diagrams to illustrate the different massaging techniques. He took one look at the paper and said, "Porn!" I knew he was on board.

It took 40 minutes for him to get through some of the massages, and we didn't even finish them all. The said exercises were to be completed in three sets of five, which was a lot of massaging. Afterward, I thought I would try to read before bed. One problem. My husband had massaged my boobs for 40 minutes. He had other things on his mind, and I was certainly game for his idea. The book could wait for tomorrow.

The following morning, I drove myself into town. I arrived at the mastectomy store. The sales associate recognized me and smiled. I asked if she received my prescription. She said, "No, but don't worry. We're going to get you set up. If the prescription doesn't show up in a few days, I'll give you a call." Then she asked what I needed. I pulled out the catalog and showed her the padding.

She took me into her private room and pulled out a gray colored pad. It looked like a maxi pad for someone the size of King Kong. We shoved the padding into the Spanx-like compression bra, and I could barely get it closed.

I turned and looked in the mirror. I felt like a little girl playing dress up with one of my mom's bras, but the little girl overstuffed the bra with a bunch of dad's socks. It was so lumpy. I guess my expression was enough to make the sales associate roar with laughter. She said, "You can wear this at night. Don't worry about trying to wear it all the time." We chuckled at the thought of walking out of this store with lumpy breasts.

My first night with the padding stuffed inside my compression bra was so exciting. Not really. It was even less sexy than wearing the compression bra. I didn't care how I looked because I was sure by tomorrow morning the right jug would have deflated like a Tom Brady football. Unfortunately, it didn't deflate at all; in fact, I think it was worse.

I pressed my hand up against my right breast. It felt like a softball had moved in under the skin. It was no longer the squishy, gel-like implant, and I panicked. What first? Dial 911, or my plastic surgeon. I talked myself off the ledge and decided to give her a little love. I massaged both boobs as my physical therapist taught me. Wax on, wax off. Wax on, wax off. Then I put on a clean and sexy compression bra without the King Kong sized maxi pad and went about my day. I reminded myself that this was another part of the battle. The Troublemaker had been traumatized and she needed some time to heal. Patience.

Four days with my fancy new contraption and nothing. The girls were swollen and the right side full. It was a constant reminder; multiple lymph nodes were fired from their post and there were only a few remaining who were working very hard to help pick up the slack without overtime pay.

I started my morning massage routine telling my lymph nodes that it was okay to share the responsibility. I was literally talking to my boobs and my lymph nodes. I assured my right lady lymph nodes that they were among friends. I told them to let go of the swelling and let all her friends help.

When I was about three quarters of the way through my boob massage, Adlai peeked his head in the door, "How are things going?" he asked. "Do you need me to do anything?"

I replied with a frustrated, "No." He sat down next to me on the bed. Tears hung along edges of my eyelids. I blinked and felt the cool salty tear roll down my cheek. "I feel like it's not working. I don't understand why they had to take so many lymph nodes especially if I have to go through chemotherapy."

He plucked a tissue from the Kleenex box on my nightstand. He wiped the streaming tears away and held me close to his chest. He was warm and comforting and told me this was a journey. "It won't be this way forever. You still have three full weeks with the physical therapist before chemo starts," he said. "Talk to her on Tuesday and ask her if this is normal. Ask her how long she thinks it will take."

"I am done with this," I said. "What if it takes six months?" I asked.

"Then it'll take six months," he said. "Come on, let's go for a walk. I think you need some fresh air."

I gathered myself, and we walked the streets around the golf course across from our house. The sun was warm; the wind was strong, but pleasant. We talked about the beautiful deciduous trees. It was late summer in Minnesota and there were three trees in our neighborhood that had fiery red, rusty orange, and bright golden yellow leaves fluttering on the spiny tree branches. By the time we returned home I had forgotten about my swollen, firm boob.

During a chat with my dear friend, Beverly, she encouraged me to try yoga. She said the breathing would be relaxing, and some of the stretches may prove helpful for strengthening and lengthening the axillary cording in my right armpit.

Later that day, I went downstairs to my workout studio and pulled up a beginner Vinyasa yoga video on YouTube. It was 20 minutes, and I loved it. This was an aberration. I hate yoga. I have tried it over and over, and I have always thought it was the most useless workout a person could ever do. Relax. Who needed to relax? Time was of the essence, and if I was going to spend an hour working out, I was going to feel it.

When I finished the workout, I found some meditation music and meditated for about 15 minutes. Or tried to meditate. My go-to meditation techniques were running, journaling, and coloring. Either one of these allowed me to let go of thoughts and enjoy the moment. Each was rhythmic and expressive in its own way. While running outside, I would take in all the colors of nature and the act of writing or coloring always mesmerized me.

During my first meditation session, I broke concentration on my breath and reminded my right lymph nodes that being short staffed didn't need to be debilitating. The lymphatic system was far-reaching, and it was a powerhouse. I settled back to my breath. Inhale. Exhale. Inhale. Exhale. I added yoga and meditation to my daily ritual.

The following Tuesday morning, I had another PT appointment. She spent several minutes pressing and pulling on cording in my armpit. As she worked, she reminded me to breathe throughout the session. Each time I exhaled and relaxed, I felt the cording relax and lengthen. After the session, I mentioned I had done yoga the day before. She was shocked. At first, I thought she was going to scold me. But her response was quite the contrary. She praised me and said, "Did you practice the breathing technique with the yoga poses?"

"Of course," I said. Then I told her about the breathing and meditation afterward.

She praised me again. "Controlled breathing during yoga and meditation affects the right side of your lymphatic system. It's one of the best things you can do for your situation," she said.

My daily routine became a new adventure. Each day was filled with finger walking, breast massages, long walks, yoga, and meditation. Sometimes while I was out for a walk, I would reminisce about the high intensity workouts I used to do. I remembered all the miles I put on each year pounding the pavement, plowing through multiple pairs of tennis shoes every year. I enjoyed this new path I was on. It was different, intriguing. I liked learning and practicing new things. It was a long-awaited overhaul for my mind, body, and soul.

On my third physical therapy appointment, I walked in to the same small, private room searching for strength, begging myself to withhold the emotions that were bubbling up. My therapist closed the door. She asked me to remove my top and compression bra. My chest tightened, and my eyes burned. I could bathe in the tears that spewed from my eyes.

"What's wrong?" my physical therapist asked. My chest heaved and a lump in my throat blocked any words from exiting my mouth. I tried desperately to tell her about my day with the oncologist.

I stood by her in the small room, boobs exposed. A chill ran down my spine. Half-naked and sobbing she embraced me. She told me I was in a safe place. "You can cry as long as you need to. Share when you are ready," she said softly. In between chest heaves I apologized again and again.

"I...I...I" I stuttered, chest heaving. "I had my...my...first" I hesitated and heaved again. I finally spoke in one sentence as she encouraged me to breathe.

"My first appointment with my oncologist was today," I said. "I only have a couple more weeks with you before chemo starts. I read that chemo and radiation make the axillary cording worse, and there's a big chance lymphedema will occur, and I am going into menopause," I cried.

"Okay, first of all, I will not dismiss you as a patient until we have you healed. We'll get more sessions booked today." She said. "For now, lie down and let's work through this."

I cried for the entire hour. It was pitiful. As she massaged my sternum and chest, I could feel three short, sharp heaves. Then I would take a big deep breath. Again, three short, sharp heaves. Big deep breath. I was horrified, embarrassed, and terrified at the next phase of my treatment.

# Part 3: Chemotherapy

# Poison Control

I had met with my oncologist three hours before that embarrassing physical therapy appointment—the one where I sobbed the entire hour. For two hours I listened and absorbed information from my oncologist while damming a tidal wave of tears sitting behind my eyelids.

My oncologist was an attractive man in a nerdy kind of way. He had a dark olive complexion with rosy cheeks and jet-black hair perfectly coiffed with a light gel. His square black framed glasses slipped down the bridge of his nose every few minutes, so he used his middle finger to push his glasses up. "What do you know about your upcoming chemotherapy journey?" he asked me.

I responded with a confidence. "There are three reasons why I have to have chemo," I said. "First, I had two tumors removed, second, one was larger than one centimeter, and finally, cancer was in my lymph nodes."

"Those variables play a part in why you are having chemo," he said, "but there's more to this phase."

I wasn't prepared for this response. I wasn't expecting any more bombs to be dropped; unfortunately, my oncologist had a different plan of attack. "One of the main reasons we chose the path I am recommending is because we believe the second tumor was actually a lymph node and the cancer was trying to break out of the node," he said. "We rated your cancer as Stage 3."

I felt like I had been zapped with a taser. The thought of strong and fierce lymph nodes being too weak for the disease inside of me left me stunned, speechless. Cancer was trying to host a party in the rest of my precious cargo. It never occurred to me that the cancer could have spread beyond the lymph nodes.

Nicole L. Czarnomski

My oncologist explained two different chemotherapy options. The first drug was called Paclitaxel, or Taxol, and it would be administered every third week for three months. This option was aggressive. "This treatment is brutal on the nerves in your fingertips and toes. It can kill the cells and they will not regenerate. This is called neuropathy," he explained.

The second option was two months of an aggressive concoction including Cytoxan and Adriamycin. Then three months of Taxol only in lighter doses as not to kill off those nerve endings. In total: five months of chemotherapy.

He recommended the five-month option because the side effects weren't as difficult. The second option did have some hideous side effects, but because I was young, I would have an easier time coping with the drugs. One of the drugs in option two affected the heart. Prior to treatment, I would undergo an echocardiogram to make sure my ticker was strong and healthy.

"If you were 80 years old, I would hesitate to recommend this drug, but because you are young and seemingly healthy, I think this will be okay," he said.

He went on to discuss the second and third part of my treatment plan. Radiation was the second step and would be administered every day for approximately one month. Each treatment would last 20-30 minutes. The last step was an oral medication called Tamoxifen. This drug would shut down my ovaries and limit the amount of hormones racing through my body. This was known as hormone replacement therapy or endocrine therapy. The reason for the hormone blocking treatment was because the type of cancer I had was hormone based. I was ER positive (estrogen) and PR positive (progesterone). This drug would initiate menopause.

I was prepared for the chemo discussion, but the news about radiation and menopause in my early 40s left me slumped over in my chair, eyes staring at my feet. This news was as shocking to learn as the Space Shuttle Challenger exploding while sitting in fifth grade science class back in January of 1986. Shocking and devastating.

As he talked, my mind wandered. Anger inundated my thoughts. I was angry at the doctor who said the American Cancer Society recommended mammograms at age 45 instead 40 for women with no history of breast cancer in their family. I was furious with her for not telling me birth control pills could cause cancer. That tidbit could have altered my thought process a few years ago when she asked if I wanted to investigate other birth control options.

I started taking the pill in my early 20s because I had surgery to remove an ovarian cyst the size of a small grapefruit. The pill was supposed to help my lower lady parts stay healthy and cyst-free. But said pill screwed my upper lady parts. At least that was what I was led to believe when my general surgeon told me to stop taking them the same day he told me I had breast cancer.

My oncologist continued with a list of side effects from endocrine therapy: it could cause vaginal dryness, vaginal itching, hot flashes, irregular periods and low sex drive. Having a low sex drive made me sad. I was sad for me, but I was heartbroken for Adlai. Hasn't he been through enough? I wanted so desperately to start bringing home good news for him, news that our life was going to turn around; news that made him happy, me happy. Instead, we'd have more bad news.

Cue the fucking tears. Wasn't there a valve on the tear ducts? Like a toilet. If a toilet overflows, you simply turn it off. Maybe my tear duct valve was broken. Maybe I was born without one. Maybe it was good I didn't have one because that would be one more thing to break or get cancer.

When I asked him why I needed radiation too, he told me that I was young and needed every possible procedure to kill the cancer cells within my body. "What are the side effects of radiation?" I asked.

"I would rather you speak to your radiation oncologist when the time comes. They will be able to discuss the appropriate treatment and the effects of radiation. We are going to start with chemotherapy first," he said.

"I will think about radiation, but it seems like overkill. I don't know if I will choose radiation therapy or not," I said like it wasn't a choice between life or death.

After we discussed the entire treatment plan, he went on to reveal the side effects of chemo. I told him I had a serious aversion to throwing up. "I have emetophobia. I looked it up. It means fear of barfing. I need anything and everything to keep me from barfing," I said. He told me there were many ways to help with nausea and vomiting. Apparently, chemo drugs and anti-nausea pills have come a long way since the days of making the toilet your BFF.

My oncologist wanted to know what I was thinking about the treatment options. I decided the option that wasn't going to kill the nerves in my fingers and toes was the best one; the option that would only screw with my heart was the best choice. Another reason I chose option two was because he told me if I were his sister, he would insist on choosing it. I took his recommendation.

This plan would take me five months. The first two months were considered aggressive. I swallowed hard and listened to the remainder of his recommendations. The final three months of chemo were less aggressive but were administered every week and would wipe out my white blood cell counts.

My oncologist reminded me again, "My team and I will do everything we can to help with nausea and vomiting. During the aggressive treatments, we will also be injecting you with a drug to help elevate your white blood cells, so your immune system isn't as compromised."

He asked about my employment and financial status. I responded, "I work with the public. I am on my feet a lot. I need to work to help support my family." I contemplated returning to work in one week since I was recovering nicely after my surgery, but the look on his face told me everything.

"If possible, you will more than likely want to rest at least for the first four rounds of treatment," he said. "Dealing with the public can be exhausting and there are a lot of germs that can and will be harmful to you while you are receiving this treatment." He danced around the topic when I told him I would rest for the first four aggressive treatments and return to work when the weekly treatments started.

"Can you please explain to me again why radiation is in my treatment plan?" I asked. "I am concerned about the axillary cording in my right armpit and the implants."

"You don't have the expanders in?" He asked.

"No, my doctor went straight to implants," I replied.

"Remind me please, who is your plastic surgeon?" He asked scanning notes in the computer.

"I had my surgery at another hospital," I said.

"Again, Nicole, I feel you should discuss this with the radiation oncologist. Let's focus on the chemo for now," he said.

His response was fine with me; I didn't want to think about radiation treatment. I wanted more time to mull it over. One step at a time I thought.

Because of the runaway cancer that was found in my lymph nodes, there were several tests I had to undergo. The tests would include a CT scan of my chest, abdomen, and pelvic area, as well as a bone scan. Terror ripped through me. I couldn't believe I needed to be tested for bone cancer. That was bad. Very bad.

When I returned home after the appointment, Adlai embraced me, enveloped me in love and support. I sat down on the sofa trembling in fear, shaking like a California earthquake.

The following morning, I had back to back appointments at the clinic for tests to determine if the cancer had moved into other parts of my body. At 6:30 a.m., I waited in line for my first blood draw, then ambled to my next appointment and waited for an injection to assist with the bone scan. After these two appointments, I waited to be prepped for a CT scan.

I had two hours before my CT scan, so I sat in the waiting room trying to read my book. Each word rear-ended the other word causing a massive traffic jam on each page. Because of these appointments, I was not allowed to drink coffee or eat breakfast, two things that help get my motor started each morning. Exhaustion and stress plagued my body.

As my eyelids drooped and my head bobbed, I felt someone creep up next to me. It was a dear friend offering a hug. I smiled. She sat with me and chatted for about 20 minutes, and for a few moments, she took my mind off cancer.

Finally, at 10:20 a.m. my pager went off. It was my turn. The nurse put the IV in my right arm and was kind enough to wrap it with gauze when she saw me cringe at the needle. She led me into a room with a large machine for the CT scan. The technician had me lay face up. She asked me to raise my right arm up over my head.

My arm went up, and I winced. "Higher please," she said when I couldn't lift my arm any further. Exhausted and stressed I barked, "I can't lift it any higher. There is axillary cording in my armpit restraining my arm. I had 18 lymph nodes removed on this side! Didn't you read my chart? I just had a double mastectomy, and I am still healing."

The activity in the room came to a stop. There was an eerie silence. I felt like a person dying on the emergency room table. There were no voices, only a white light. And then the chaos ensued.

"No, we aren't privy to this information. We are only told to run the scan," the tech said. "Has anyone told you not to use your right arm for IVs, needle sticks, and blood pressure checks?" she asked.

"No, no one has told me any of this!" I growled again.

"I'm sorry, we're going to get the nurse," the tech said to me.

The nurse came in and apologized. She said, "We have to put the IV in the left arm." Heat surged through my body, my face flushed and punching someone felt like an appropriate reaction. I maintained composure and faced my fear of needles as needle number four made its way into my left vein in the crease of my elbow.

After the IV was in my left arm, I was prepped for the scan. They described the sensation I was about to feel as the liquid from the IV was injected into my body. "This injection will feel like you are wetting your pants. You aren't, but you will feel a warm sensation in that area," she said.

The nurse pushed the liquid into the IV site, and 20 seconds later, I could feel the heat. It was like warm pee flooded the lower half of my body. Then, as quickly as it came, it left, and a cool sensation overcame my whole body giving me the chills.

When the CT scan was completed, I had five minutes to get to my next appointment in another building. One of the nurses fetched a wheelchair, a warm blanket and a $10 gift certificate to eat in the cafeteria for the stressful situation I experienced. She took me through the staff hallways and elevators so I would arrive at my next appointment on time.

It was time for the bone scan, and the nurse pulled both IV needles from my arm and set me up in the machine. She strapped me down on a large platform and told me to lie still. Nothing sounded better than lying down and doing nothing. If only I were at the beach sipping on a cocktail.

When the bone scan was completed, I was tired and wanted them to keep searching so I could drift to sleep. It was only a breath away, and I wanted a moment of peace. The technicians were oblivious to my desires and helped me out of the machine. The tests were complete. Now the waiting game. My next appointment was with my oncologist, but I had time to go get something to eat.

I found the cafeteria, and I picked out a chicken salad sandwich, chips, nuts, a bottle of water and grapes. I wanted to spend every cent on the gift certificate. I wished coffee could have been included in lunch, but I was instructed to consume water to flush my system; I had to wait for my savory dark cup of coffee for another day.

Nicole L. Czarnomski

Although I needed sustenance, the food didn't seem to fill the void. I picked at the sandwich like a bird, as I imagined cancer writhing throughout my body. Where had I gone wrong? Why was I the chosen one? Breast cancer. Cancer in the lymph nodes. Now, cancer could be holed up in another part of my precious body. Why me?

After tossing most of the food in the garbage wondering where my appetite went, I walked to my final appointment. What was waiting on the other side of the doorway? I sat in a chair in the waiting room and let my head bob up and down. I dozed off and on for a couple of hours until my pager went off. The results loomed in the computer database with hundreds of thousands of other patients.

My oncologist burst into the room with a victorious voice, "You are free and clear. We didn't see anything unusual at all in the test we ran. Congratulations!"

Temporary relief. Now, I could focus on the looming months ahead. He scheduled an appointment for an echocardiogram the following week along with an appointment with my nurse educator who would be providing vital information about my upcoming chemotherapy.

The day was over, so I called Adlai and asked him to pick me up. He arrived a few minutes later and drove me home. That night, sleep came easily. At 10 the next morning, I managed to rise and get on with my day, though my thoughts were inundated with chemo, vomiting, hair loss, radiation, and more time off work. How would I manage this next phase? Staying positive, keeping a high frequency with the Universe by doing yoga, meditating, writing, and walking were the recipe for success.

Nicole L. Czarnomski

Before my first chemo appointment, I met with the nurse
educator. As I made my way up the elevator to the waiting room, fear
tore through my mind and body. It ran deep in my worn-out veins. It
sliced through any thoughts I had of being a warrior. Chemotherapy felt
like my death sentence.

Rachel, the nurse educator, saved me from the thunderstorm of
thoughts roiling around in my brain. Her voice was soft and kind. Her
face was round and her eyes blue. Everything about her was genuine
and helpful. I was astounded at the available resources to help make
chemo manageable.

Rachel brought booklets and pamphlets that discussed every
side effect and issue cancer and chemo caused. Carrying a backpack
today would have been a smart move, but alas I only had my small
purse so I would schlep all the material in my arms, hugging my chest.

We spent an hour and half going through every piece of
literature. Rachel educated me on proper nutrition, food preparation,
exercise, sex and sexuality, grief, counseling, and loss. The clinic
provided free classes for nutrition, stress management, art classes,
Reiki and healing touch classes, symptom management, breathing and
meditation sessions multiple times per week. She said there were
additional floors built onto the clinic's fitness center for public use.
This new center offered meditation, spa services, and a quiet place to
hang out. Chemo seemed less horrific at this point.

She saw the tension in my face lighten and a smile cross my
face. That was when she hit me with the disclaimer, "Chemo isn't going
to be a walk in the park, Nicole, but we are here to try to make it a little
easier. You shouldn't feel miserable for five straight months."

We discussed my vomiting phobia. Emetophobia. I chose not
to use the term emetophobia, because I figured most people were not
aware of the formal name associated with this terrible disease. She

smiled and said, "Make sure to let your doctor know. He will take good care of you. We don't want you throwing up either because it causes dehydration."

During this meeting, she also gave me helpful tips. She said, "Put the on-call phone number into your phone contact list along with the main clinic number so you have it with you wherever you go. Then, make sure you can access to the online portal for ease in communication. Use this to ask questions and reschedule appointments."

After meeting with Rachel, I was actually excited to start chemo because of all the resources I had at my fingertips. Perhaps Rachel should be in sales. I think she would do a fine job. Maybe that was her secret title. Maybe she was the chemo salesperson. I bet she won the award last year for best chemo salesperson of the year. I hope it was a nice prize.

# Chemo Party

After I learned my chemo schedule, my Fitness Friends hosted a chemo party. A party for chemo may sound odd, but trust me, it was a good thing. We gathered one evening at Sarah's house. We ate, talked, and laughed. I enjoyed the food that night like a hiker who had traversed a 14er with nothing more than a few dried fruits and nuts. I knew food may be an issue in the coming months, so I savored every bite.

The party took my buzzing mind off the looming chemotherapy treatments. My friend Kellie brought her five-week-old baby. I was not a baby person because I felt like I might break them. Their little heads bobbled around, and they made me nervous. Plus, they might poop, vomit, or sneeze and that was out of my comfort zone. However, the little bundle brought innocence and hope to that party; she made me giddy.

The infant was passed around like a bong at a frat house. Everyone wanted a piece of the innocence, not wanting to give her up to the next person. I sat in awe checking out the tiny little toes and toenails. She was beautiful and perfect.

The food line started with me. I filled my plate like it was the last supper, and I walked out to the patio to sit down. It was a gorgeous fall evening. The sun warmed the back of head, my hair blowing gently in the wind. As we ate, we went around the table, so everyone had their chance to give life updates. We discussed vacations, jobs, childbirth, and so many beautiful things we had going in life. Laughter filled the air, and for the first time in a while, I was happy. Happy to have been given another day on the planet with so many beautiful women by my side.

I burned each moment in my mind to carry with me when things were difficult. Learning to savor each moment and learning to be grateful for everything was a part of this journey. I had heard cancer changes your life. It was true. It made me slow down and be grateful; my life was filled with many positive things.

Seven weeks passed since my original boobs were taken from me. Gone forever. One of the very things that made me a woman. Gone in a five-hour surgery. For the last several weeks, I went to physical therapy and had seen small improvements. Boob-a-dema was less of an issue, and the axillary cording had started to ease. Shaving my right armpit was not easy. I was no longer allowed to use a razor blade because the microscopic cuts from the blade could lead to an infection, so I used an electric razor. Shaving with a giant cord running through the pit was not easy. The electric razor left uneven sprouts of hair growing from my armpit. The razor merely grazed on the hair like a hungry cow in the pasture. Maybe I needed to spend more than 30 dollars on an electric razor, but it seemed like a reasonable amount to do the job.

I decided to check out the online forums for shaving after a mastectomy. Perhaps someone had found an electric razor that worked. In reading forums, I found some people weren't following directions. Some women said they continued to use their beautiful Gillette Venus razors on their armpits without any problems.

When it came to anything medical, I was a rule follower, so I didn't want to take any chances. An infection sounded gnarly. I continued to follow the rules, and I used my razor that left stubble to gather sweat underneath my armpits. Pew! Sweaty armpits.

Nicole L. Czarnomski

With my armpit woes fresh in my mind, I left the house ready for my first chemo treatment, or as ready as I could be. I chose to continue my leave of absence at work until after my aggressive chemo was complete, and on September 28, 2017 my veins and body were flooded with the first round of the Adriamycin and Cytoxan cocktail.

Adlai parked in the lot across from the clinic. As we climbed up, up, up on the concrete parking structure, my face tightened and started to tingle. My lips were dry, and I could feel a lump forming in my throat.

We walked to the waiting room. The receptionist asked my name, "Nicole Czarnomski, C-Z," I said.

"Oh, that's helpful, I would have typed a Z," she said. She passed a translucent, maroon pager across the desk and told me to have a seat. My butt barely reached the chair when the pager went off signaling me it was time for the blood test. I wished I had taken an Ativan to melt the icy snowball in my throat. I had to complete blood work first to ensure my white blood cell count was high enough to withstand the upcoming drugs.

The second vibration from my pager startled me. I was cleared for chemo. Adlai and I walked toward the doorway of the chemo ward. Dani stood at the entryway and introduced herself. She was dressed in all black except a pale blue shirt underneath her black sweater. She was happy and sweet, and I appreciated her smile. She asked me to remove my shoes, take off my jacket, and set my handbag down to obtain the correct height and weight. This was a critical step that determined how the chemo cocktail was prepared. Chemo was custom-made for every patient.

I walked by multiple rooms with other cancer patients lying down with tubes sticking out of their arms. As we rounded the corner, a patient met us. The woman was walking with her medications in tow.

She had a tube sticking out of her arm and it was attached to bags hooked on a tall skinny wheeled cart. I cringed at the sight, knowing it would soon be me.

Dani walked us to my private room. The neighboring rooms had their curtains open and patients were sitting up in their chairs chatting with friends and family members and watching television. Very few were in beds resting quietly. I hoped I wasn't going to be the latter.

After she showed us my room, Dani took us to the snack lounge. It was loaded with lots of yummy food and drinks. "Help yourself to as much as you want," she smiled before showing us back to my room. My room had a heated massage chair that I activated immediately. It was like the chairs at the nail salon. For one moment I fantasized about pedicures, but then the nurse arrived with a needle.

They didn't waste any time prepping me for treatment. I bragged about how awesome my veins were to get my mind off chemo. In the past, I have had so many nurses tell me my veins are easy to hit. A look of pride crossed my face. I took off my jacket and I showed the nurse my arm. "See?" I said, pointing to my arm. "Awesome, huh?"

"Well, I'm actually going to put this needle in the top of your hand."

Curses, I thought. I remember the last IV placed in my hand was when I had my boobs sliced off. The IV site hurt for days after surgery. That's all I could think about now as he pulled the rubber tourniquet around my arm. He tapped my hand. He tapped it again. He knew I was getting nervous and asked if I was afraid of needles.

"Uh huh," I managed to whimper. He assured me that it would be over shortly. He asked if I wanted to know when the needle was going in. "Yes! Yes, I want to know!" I thought it was a requirement

94

Nicole L. Czarnomski

for nurses to inform the patient of the "little stick and a burn." Maybe not? He let me know and the needle went in. "Awesome. We're good, right?" I asked.

"I can't tell. I might have missed," he said. I thought he was joking until he kept tapping it. Like a balloon deflating, I blew out all the air I was holding in my chest. The word fell out of my mouth. "Fuuucckk." It wasn't directed at him. It wasn't loud or forceful or mean, just deflated and encumbered by stress. This guy may need to re-stick my arm. I needed Rachel to sell me on this chemo thing again because of this stupid needle. I wondered if she was a needle salesperson too.

I was scratching my right leg so hard with my opposite hand, Adlai had to stop me and remind me it was only a needle. He looked at me with his big brown eyes and sweet smile and said, "You've got this. Come on. It's only a needle. This is the easiest part."

Today, it was more than a needle. Poison was on the other side of that needle waiting to wriggle inside my body into the deepest, darkest crevice to mold to every cell available, good or bad. I had no idea what side effects this poison would have besides the ones already discussed. There could be more unknown darkness lying within this needle.

My nurse left my room and returned with another nurse. She tapped the location a few times and said, "Perfect." Those words were magical and terrifying. I had done it. I survived the needle stick, but now it was time for the Red Devil, the chemo, the poison.

The Red Devil was a term coined by the chemo team. The drug's real name was Adriamycin. The drug itself was red and gave patients red pee for a few days after treatment. This drug caused hair loss, nausea and vomiting, decreased white blood cell and platelet

95

counts, mouth sores, skin redness and itching and irritation at the injection site.

When my dose had been prepared, the nurse entered my room with a large syringe. She was cloaked in a blue, papery smock and wore rubber gloves. If her skin was exposed to the drug, it could literally burn the flesh. "Do you like Popsicles?" She asked. I thought it was a strange question, but I took the bait.

"Sure!" I said.

"What flavor?" She asked.

"Red, I guess," still wondering why she was asking about popsicles.

Another nurse entered my room and was instructed to fetch a red Popsicle. As the nurse went to retrieve the Popsicle, the nurse prepping the Red Devil said it was a good idea to suck on something cold to numb the nerve endings in my mouth. "This is a way to prevent mouth sores," she said.

My red Popsicle arrived the same time the Red Devil was thrust into my veins for the very first time. With this drug, the nurse had to push the entire amount from the syringe into my body because if any poison escapes the vein or if there was redness at the site, tissue could be burned and damaged. I had to put a lot of trust in the nurse pushing the Red Devil.

We talked about getting my head shaved. I had scheduled an appointment on October 2, but she recommended waiting another week. She said, "Hair loss happens after three or four weeks. You might as well keep that long beautiful, brown hair another week."

After the Red Devil had been administered, I was given the second drug. They injected me with Cytoxan which also caused nausea, vomiting, hair loss, decreased white blood cell and platelet counts, poor appetite and a metallic taste on my tongue. This was injected through an IV drip.

I watched droplets of clear fluid flow into the tube attached to my arm hoping it was targeting cancer and not all the good cells in my body, but I knew chemo worked differently. It targeted everything in its path, good or bad.

While I was waiting, my friend Denise came to visit me. She was a welcome sight. She was a yoga instructor and had the most calming, beautiful voice that could make any stress or trauma melt away. She also brought a beautiful chenille blanket with a damask pattern and a journal for me. I always loved starting a new journal. It was the perfect resting spot for fresh new stories and journal entries. I hugged her and thanked her. She stayed with Adlai and me for quite a while. She said that her friend Jodi, who was a talented hair stylist, would be happy to help me if I needed to have a wig styled. I felt grateful again for Denise and her thoughtful gestures.

As I thought of Jodi, I remembered an event she hosted at her salon, in October 2012. I participated in the Hello Gorgeous 5K with my Fitness Friend Katie and a few other friends. Jodi and Hello Gorgeous, an organization that provided complimentary makeovers to women battling all cancers, provided Red Carpet treatment to a woman with cancer while the participants dressed in cocktail dresses walked or ran a 5K. How ironic some five years later I would be the one needing the spa treatment and complimentary makeover.

About two hours later, when both drugs had been administered, the first nurse returned and attached a small device the shape of a floss dispenser to my abdomen. It had a sticky patch on it that adhered to the skin. I had to wear this device for 27 hours after my treatment. At the 27-hour mark, this device was going to pump me full of Neulasta, a man-made form of a protein that stimulated the growth of white blood cells.

She put the patch on my belly. There was some beeping and blinking and a small needle was injected into my skin—thankfully I couldn't see this needle. Once the needle made it into my skin, a tiny tube was inserted into my abdomen. The tube waited there until it was safe to pump my body with the Neulasta fluid.

The following day I took my cocktail of pills as directed. There were steroid pills and anti-nausea medications. I dozed off and on throughout the day, and I waited for my Neulasta shot. Twenty-seven hours later, the beeping commenced and within 45 minutes, all the Neulasta in the floss-shaped container was injected into my body. I looked at the contraption on my belly and the display screen showed the device as empty, so I pulled the patch off and put it in a Ziploc bag so I could dispose of it at the clinic during my next treatment. The nurse said not to dispose of this in the trash at home.

I had more energy than I thought I would. I was nauseous a few times but took the prescribed medications that worked brilliantly, allowing me to eat normally. And yes, I did pee a little bit of pink for a day or two following treatment. I was hoping for more excitement. The Red Devil didn't impress me yet.

Nicole L. Czarnomski

# Miss Buzzy vs. G.I Jane

Hair was an enigma to me. In the past four decades, I have
been a natural blonde (childhood), a bottle blonde (once my childhood
blonde hair turned mousy), a red head, and a brunette. I have had
extremely long hair, medium length hair, bobs, and pixie cuts. I have
had bangs, and I have grown out bangs dozens of times, but never have
I been bald. Even as an infant, I had a few golden locks atop my head.

I have changed hairstyles over and over to recreate a new me,
but I had never really been happy with my hair. Was it because I had
never been truly happy with who I was, or was it really just about the
hair? Did I let hair define me? Did I hide behind it?

Back in my late twenties, I yearned to be super hip, to be
someone I was not. I considered myself an artist. Day after day, I left
my day job in product development and came home each evening and
painted abstract art compositions wearing my paint splattered overalls.
At the time, I was living on the outskirts of Boston. I hadn't found a
hairdresser yet, so I picked an Aveda Salon and made an appointment.
When I arrived, the stylist sat me down and asked those dreaded words,
"So what are we doing today?"

"Just do something edgy," I said looking at myself in the
mirror. I was bored of wearing the same khaki chinos and black t-shirts
I purchased from The Gap, and I was tired of my silky, smooth blonde
hair. I hoped she had something fun that would inspire me to go out,
get a new wardrobe, and become someone else. She sold me on a new
color technique she saw at the most recent hair show in New York.

I walked out of the salon with the top part of my hair the
brightest shade of platinum I had ever seen. The bottom portion dark
brown. It was literally two-tone. I looked like a skunk when I put my
hair in a ponytail. My long, beautiful, healthy hair was so damaged

from the process I thought it might fall out. I tried not to care because the style was straight off the runways in the early 2000s. That made me hip, right? No, it just made me mad at myself for trying to take on a new persona. I hated my hair. And I still didn't like the girl hiding beneath it.

There were more bad hair days than good in my life including days I was too tired to put forth the effort to style it. Even if I did spend the time, I had no idea what to do with my hair. I had never invested in expensive curling irons or flat irons. I only used a blow dryer, a paddle or a round brush and cheap hairspray. I had clips and pins and all sorts of rubber bands, but I mostly swept it up into a ponytail or a bun.

Unlike most people, when I realized I was going to lose my hair during chemo, I felt relieved. I was elated to start over, to know what color my natural hair was. I knew it would be tough living in Minnesota during the winter without my long, thick, hair to keep my noggin warm, but I didn't care. I wrapped my brain around this thought and surprised myself when people kept asking me if I was going to get a wig. Without hesitation, I said no every time. I couldn't be bothered to care for my own hair, let alone a wig. Maybe I was lazy.

My first thought was of "G.I. Jane" and the haircut Demi Moore rocked in that movie. That simple buzz cut looked so easy to style. But then I realized I wasn't Demi Moore. What was my bald head going to look like? What if it my head was misshapen? What if I was a cone head? Was my hair hiding a cone shaped head all along? Maybe the new cut would be cute and not tough. I didn't have the punk rocker look or attitude, though I think I would choose that as my alter ego. Clearly, there was a lot of anticipation prior to the day I shaved my head.

When I called my stylist Corey to have my head shaved, I didn't speak directly to her. I called like it was any old appointment and scheduled the buzz cut. I owned it. I even told the lady on the phone, "I have cancer and I need my head shaved."

I was surprised when my friend Katie sent me a message asking if I was sure I wanted to get my head shaved alone. She had just come back from getting her hair done and Corey, my stylist, told her I had already set up my appointment for a random day at 1 p.m. I wrote back, "I don't want to bother anyone. It's just hair."

Katie told me Corey wanted to do the cut after work hours with my friends. I thought that sounded like fun, but again I thought, oh jeez, I don't want anyone to go to any trouble. Little did I know this wasn't about anyone going to any trouble, this was about a rockin' good time surrounded by people I loved. Surrounded by people who didn't care if I was bald, blonde, brunette, or a red head.

Every Monday, Aspasia Salon and Spa closed early. We scheduled my buzz cut for 5:30 p.m. Monday, October 9, 2017. There was plenty of time for friends who worked until 5 p.m. to get to the salon after work. To my surprise, several of my Fitness Friends and my husband wanted to come and support me on this occasion.

My friend Sarah picked me up a little after 5 p.m. and asked how I was doing. I told her I had been doing much better until today. "Sarah, I am getting my head shaved. When I cry you must cry with me," I said wondering what happened to the confidence I previously had about shaving my head.

When we arrived at the salon, several people were already there. Once again, my friends made this appointment a party by bringing snacks and beverages. I hugged each one of them and thanked them for coming and again said to them, "WHEN I cry, you must cry with me." Why was getting my hair buzzed suddenly a big deal?

We started with a before picture outside with of all my friends. A picture with me and my long brown hair, hair I had finally grown to love. Yes, I loved it. Last year, when Corey changed my color from blonde to brunette I fell in love with my hair. It figures—I had finally found my perfect hair and now it was about to disappear. Many people had told me that hair comes back curly, and often a different color after chemo. I had no idea what to expect next year when it grew back. I would have to deal with that later. For now, it was time to say good-bye.

My friends Ann and Sarah waited with me after the last photo. The last photo of me with hair. They hovered around me like a helicopter parent waiting for me to cry so they could comfort me. I think they could sense my hesitation and my sadness. Tears were pushing up to the surface and they both told me it was okay to be upset. It was okay to cry. They reminded me that I was embarking on another difficult phase of this journey.

I pulled myself together, and we walked back inside. Everyone was standing around having snacks and enjoying themselves. They acted like it was any old party, not a party where a girl loses the best hair she's ever had because of cancer. It was almost 6 p.m. and I knew I needed to pull myself together and go for it. I clapped my hands a few times and said, "Let's get this party started!"

The room went quiet, like a hunter who had called in his prey, waiting for it to move closer and closer before the jarring BAM! of the kill shot. I held my head up, stifled the tears and I sat down in the chair. Corey braided two pigtails tightly at the base of my neck. I wanted to get the most out of my hair so I could donate it.

Corey took out a buzz cutter because my hair was too thick to cut with scissors. Moments later, I was holding two 6-inch braids in my hand. Then Corey started to buzz the back. Hair was falling to the ground like snow in a Minnesota blizzard. As I watched it fall

Nicole L. Czarnomski

happiness overcame any sadness I was feeling. I had a room full of love surrounding me and losing my hair was not the end of the world. It would grow back. For today, I was grateful to spend time with my husband and friends, and I was grateful for their support.

My hairdresser stopped mid-shave and asked if anyone wanted to take part in the process. One by one, my friends stepped up and shaved a chunk of my hair off. Soon there was nothing left but stubble. It was liberating. I had purchased a cute pair of hoop earrings at Target that day to make the bald style look more feminine. I loved the new look! In a way, I felt tough. I felt like a Rock-n-Roll Star that could withstand any amount of poison subjected to my body. On the other hand, I felt cute and fun and sassy with the new look, like you could call me Miss Buzzy. When I looked into the mirror, I realized I wasn't either of those people. I wasn't a rock star or Miss Buzzy. I was Nicole with a nicely shaped head and the confidence to rock this new haircut. Acceptance was a beautiful thing.

# Behind Closed Doors

With all the parties and support surrounding me day in day out, it was easy to think my life was one big ball of fun despite the cancer diagnosis. In a way, yes, it had been, and I had my friends and family to thank for that. They turned every milestone into a celebration. Despite all the merriment during the weeks following my first few chemo treatments, I discovered dark places inside my mind and faced daunting physical changes I never imagined.

The Red Devil was administered every two weeks. Round two with the Red Devil was when I noticed hair loss. Even though my head was shaved, there was stubble there, and it continued to fall out.

Hair loss didn't stop at my head, it wracked my entire body. My pubic hair fell out, making me look like a 10-year-old girl. I lost the peach fuzz on my face, my eyelashes, my eyebrows, and my nose hairs. One evening before bed, Adlai ran his hand across my cheeks and gave me a soft kiss on the lips and said, "You'll always be my Sweet Peaches." As I pulled away, I started to cry. He had called me his Sweet Peaches from the day I met him because of the hair on my face. It was soft and blonde and in the right lighting was incredibly thick. I took a moment to be grateful for him and his support. I was now bald, weak, nauseous, and dizzy, but his support never once waned.

The steroids the oncologist prescribed messed up my sleep patterns and posed a threat to my heart. I was instructed to take two steroid pills for three days after each chemo treatment. This was supposed to combat fatigue, but it did its job too well. I tossed and turned every night I took them. While lying awake, I listened to my heart pounding in my chest. The heart palpations made me scared for my life. I laid awake thinking about the cancer, thinking about the chemo, thinking about the heart palpitations wondering what effects I would have long term. Oddly, I never once considered asking my doctor if I could forgo the steroids.

Around 1 a.m. for the three nights following each treatment I got up and sat on the couch devouring shows on Netflix or reading a book. As I sat slouched on the sofa, I could feel my heart pumping against my rib cage. Prior to cancer, my resting heart rate was usually 72 beats per minute, but my heart rate while on steroids increased the beats to 98 per minute. It was a change I literally felt inside me.

By 7 a.m. for three mornings following each chemo injection, I was still wide awake and would go on walks. I resisted running because it was a false sense of energy, and I didn't want to hurt myself. My body was already being beaten down with an aggressive form of chemo, so there was no sense in making it work harder.

After the steroids wore off, I was weak and tired. I couldn't do yoga, I couldn't walk, I couldn't read books because I couldn't focus. I sat on the sofa and watched television. I hated that my brain sat inside my skull wasting away. As I lounged on the sofa, my muscles felt like they were beginning to atrophy. How would I ever recover? Would I ever be the same powerhouse that I was pre-cancer?

The headaches started around day four or five. I was so nauseous I couldn't eat even after taking the anti-nausea pill; all I could do was sip on ginger ale. The lack of electrolytes coupled with the lack of food created excruciating migraines that ripped through my right eye and worked their way back on the right side of my brain.

Walking across the room was a laborious task. I would rise from the sofa in the living room to get a glass of water, and I would sit down again at the dining table and wait for another burst of energy or for a dizzy spell to disappear so I could get to the kitchen. My noggin tingled and my legs felt like they couldn't support the weight of my body. I sat at the table staring off into space waiting for the energy to get back up to try for a glass of water. Not only was I dehydrated, but the bouts of dry mouth were shocking, another side effect of chemo. Sitting at the table, I peeled back my tongue from the roof of my mouth. It felt like a dentist had left the suction tube in my mouth and then closed up shop leaving me to sit in the dental chair with no water and the tube stealing all of my saliva.

I started to feel human again about 10 days after treatments, and Adlai and I tried to take advantage of that. We were unable to have sex the first few days after treatment because of the toxicity in the Red Devil. Days four through eight left me void of any energy. Ten days out we tried to have sex, but my body was like a dried up well. One evening, our thirst for intimacy was undeniable. My patient husband took his time preparing me for the closeness we both so desired. He skillfully brought my daisy out of a wilted state, plumping her up and tenderly loving on her. Having sex was one of the best things we could have done. For me, it was a beautiful and gentle act that took my mind away from my struggles. I forgot about the large red scars running horizontally along my breasts. I forgot about being nauseous. I forgot about the headaches and dry mouth. In that moment, there was nothing but the two of us expressing our love for each other.

The following morning, I awoke around 8:30 a.m. I jolted upright as I looked at the clock. I was irritated with myself for having slept so late. I felt lazy. I reached for my robe at the end of my bed. The next thing I knew, I was on the floor holding my throbbing head. How and why was I on the floor? I rolled from my back onto my left side and grabbed the bed frame. I pressed my palm on the square bed post and pushed myself to my knees and eventually my feet. I walked to the sofa in the living room and sat down. I realized I needed to go to the bathroom. Fighting fatigue, I walked towards the bathroom leaning against the walls in the hallway. When I reached the bathroom, I sat on the edge of the tub. I opened my eyes and saw the toilet in front of me. I was confused again and wondering why I was sitting on the edge of

106

the bathtub. I made my way over to the toilet, released my bladder and was glad I was sitting on the toilet and not the sofa. I didn't think much else about the whole experience, because my mind was spacy all day and it was difficult to think.

Later in the day, I started feeling better. When Adlai returned home from work that day, I explained what happened.

"Isn't that weird?" I asked him. He looked at me strangely. I couldn't tell if he was confused or worried.

He just kept saying, "That doesn't make any sense. Why would you wake up on the floor?" Fifteen minutes later he shouted my name. He was in our bedroom. "Nicole, I think I know what happened, and I am worried."

He pointed at our wicker laundry basket. The basket had been pushed along the wall and was still standing, but there was a huge bend in the internal wire. "I think you passed out, fell into the basket and then went down on the floor. The basket broke your fall."

"Huh. I don't remember any of that. I just woke up on the floor," I said matter of fact.

"Yes, I realize that. That's why I am worried. I wasn't home. You need to be careful getting out of bed," he said. "Let me see your head. Are there any bruises?"

I rubbed my head and told him it didn't hurt anymore. There were no bumps or bruises. "How's your back? Let me see your back."

And there it was. About midway down my back a small red mark was scratched into my skin. The sore was tender, but nothing too bothersome. It was a reminder of all the things that could have happened.

I promised to get out of bed slowly. Each morning, I sat on the edge of my bed before putting my feet on the floor. I counted to 20 before standing up.

The day of my third treatment I met with my oncologist and we discussed the nasty symptoms I had. I told him about the headaches, dry mouth, sleepless nights, and weakened state. "Yes, this is chemo, and this is pretty typical. It will continue and can be more pronounced over the coming days," he said. Then I told him about fainting. He seemed perplexed when I brought this up.

"First of all, you need to be getting more electrolytes. Try drinking Gatorade," he said. I shuddered at the idea. Gatorade was like the sugar water humans mixed up and put inside hummingbird feeders. "Gross. You want me to drink sugar water?" I asked with a snarky tone.

"Yes, you need to replenish your sodium levels and Gatorade has lots of electrolytes. Looking at your blood work today, your sodium levels are low again. We need to keep those up so you don't get dehydrated. That may help with headaches too," he said. "However, the headaches are a symptom of the chemo so keep taking Tylenol for them."

He mentioned another echocardiogram because of the fainting spell. "It could be an arrhythmia that caused it," he said. He left nothing to chance and while I appreciated it, I didn't have the mental capacity to handle any more side effects or mishaps. I just wanted to get through chemo. I had battled my way through round two, and I knew it was about to become more difficult, though to what extent, I didn't know.

My pager beeped at 3:20 p.m. The clinic assistant came out of the open doors and waited for me. "Name and birthdate?" She asked. The assistant weighed me and took me to the back room next to the lounge. While the lab was preparing the Red Devil, I indulged in a Rice Krispie treat. They told me it was good to have food in my stomach or the steroids may upset it. I found it unusual the lounge offered all pre-packaged food especially since one of the cancer classes offered at the clinic was about nutrition. I was positive the pre-packaged Rice Krispie treat did not fall under healthy food items.

I tried to rev up excitement for round three. After today, I would be three quarters of the way done with the Red Devil. Another milestone. My mom was scheduled to join me today, so I had a lot to get excited about. She and my dad had made the trek from Missouri for another visit. My friends were hosting a benefit the following Sunday, and they wanted to be part of the festivities.

I was surprised to have my mom come to treatment. We both hate hospitals, and anything involved with hospitals. She arrived before the Red Devil was ready for me, so she was able to experience the whole treatment. She was so brave, and I was proud of her as she sat and watched the nurse insert the IV. This nurse was a pro who nailed it the first time. No questions about the needle stick, she simply plunged it into my hand and rolled up my arm in an electric blanket. Mom and I chatted until my first drug was ready to be injected. I'm sure my mom was less than thrilled to see poison injected into her baby girl.

The nurse brought in the Red Devil about 15 minutes later along with a couple of Popsicles, one for me and one for mom. I hadn't experienced any mouth sores, so I guess the popsicles worked. Mom and I chatted until Adlai came through the door. She surprised us both when she said my brother, T.J., and his girlfriend, Angie, were making the drive from Missouri too. T.J. and Angie would arrive on Saturday. The three of us talked until 5:45. My third round of treatment was over, and it was time to go home, where my dad was waiting with a truck full of items for the silent auction for the benefit.

For much of Saturday I napped on the sofa while mom, dad and Adlai ran errands. They returned home to another surprise: my cousin Stefani and her husband Chuck were here! They were in town for the benefit as well. We all enjoyed a light dinner Saturday night and had a great time catching up with one another.

# Benefit for My Boobs

At first, I was vehemently against a benefit, but my tribe wanted to help anyway they could. I had met my insurance deductible months ago after my surgery. The beginning of a new year was around the corner and I would be shelling out more money to meet the deductible again.

After I agreed, my friends Sarah and Brittney started planning one hell of an event. They were receiving so many silent auction items they were worried the venue would be too small and questioned whether there would be enough people to bid on all the goodies.

Silent auction donations were coming from friends, friends of friends and family members, including hubby and me. Yes, my husband and I donated several hand-made things to the auction. We had a workshop with lots of tools, and I found things on Pinterest for us to create. We bonded over sawing, nailing, gluing, and painting. Several local businesses donated items. A local liquor store even donated a bartender for the event.

The day of the benefit, my family arrived early to help the girls set up the space. They were right, there were too many donations and not enough space. Before silent auction bidding sheets could be paired with each item, people started coming through the doors. It was 12:40 p.m. and the event was supposed to start at 1 p.m. For the next two hours, it was a constant stream of people.

I tried to focus my attention on each person who arrived. I wanted to genuinely thank them for coming and to catch up with them, but the line continued to grow. It was astounding to see people lining up at the door including more of my family, my cousin Derek and his wife Lori, who made the trip from the Minneapolis/St. Paul area. There was even one very special resident from my work who attended the benefit. People waited patiently for their turn to stop and talk to me, and I later found out some people were there, but didn't get a chance to say hi.

I didn't think I knew enough people to warrant a benefit, let alone create one with such a successful outcome, though I do attribute a lot of the success to the team who hosted the event. I can't even begin to imagine the work they had to do to pull it off. And there were never going to be enough thank yous to pass along to them.

At the end of the event I was exhausted and hungry. I never had an opportunity to snack on the donated meat and cheese tray or sip on some water. I made my way over to the snack bar. As I nibbled on crackers, the girls tallied the cash and checks received at the end of the auction. The fundraiser brought in almost $4000; enough to make a significant dent in my insurance deductible. I literally stood in the middle of everyone and cried. I couldn't believe I had spent much of my adult life with low self-esteem and being overly critical of the person I had become. I was astounded thinking back to all the fitness classes I led. Me, standing in front of strong, healthy women starring in the mirror in front of me criticizing any little bit of fat I saw resting on my curvy body. What kind of example was I setting? I pushed my physical limits. I made my muscles want to ignite while they trembled through the brutal exercises. Little did I know that person I had become touched many hearts, lifted many spirits, inspired others to do their best, and was a caring friend to many. How did I not see that person? I realized at that moment there was something terribly skewed with the way I looked at and valued myself, and I knew at some point this would need to be addressed. But how? When? My job right now was to survive and thrive while going through chemo. I didn't know where to start, but I knew I would try each day to smile at the person I had become and give her as much love as I would give to my friends or my husband or to one of my family members.

Nicole L. Czarnomski

The following day, my family departed, and I was alone again. In some ways this was good, since I needed to rest, in some ways it was bad, because in my mind, despite the beauty of the weekend, things got really dark. Round three challenged my body like nothing I have ever experienced.

Like round one and two, I started with sleepless nights. The steroids pumped me up and made me feel like Super Woman. I picked a short, but intense workout DVD by a celebrity trainer. I thought it would be a great way to expend energy. It was 30 minutes, the perfect length of time. I lunged and curled and squatted with three-pound weights in each hand, feeling each muscle in my inner thighs quiver. I couldn't finish the workout. At the 22-minute mark, my body screamed stop! And the days following were not pleasant.

As a healthy person, the feeling of sore and shredded muscles was amazing, but for someone on chemo, this was detrimental to my health and well-being. My legs trembled as I squatted over the toilet. I struggled down the stairwell sideways taking each step one at a time. I hated that the laundry room was in the foyer. I ached all over. I struggled through yoga videos, so I settled for short walks.

By Wednesday, I had gotten carried away. I walked too far. I wished I would have listened to the voice that said, stop, turn around, and go home, but I didn't. I pushed too hard and then came back home and could barely move. I sat slumped on the sofa with the television on, nauseous and exhausted. I waited two hours before I had the energy to get up and get a ginger ale from the refrigerator. A migraine started late Wednesday afternoon, but I was too tired to move. I sat on the sofa in agony. If I sat still enough, I could manage the pain, and I thought I would wait it out. Big mistake. Huge.

My brain felt like someone took an ax and carved a wedge into the top of my head. Adlai returned home from work late that evening and helped me into the shower after swallowing 1000 mg of extra

113

strength Tylenol. Too weak to stand, he set up my shower chair and helped me into the bathtub. Warm water swaddled me as I hunched over. I grabbed the top of my head and rocked back and forth sobbing a weak and pitiful cry. He left me for a moment to fetch Gatorade. "Here sip some of this," his voice counseled. The cold beverage only made the pain worse. He turned off the water and pulled the soft, white towel from the bar and helped me dry off. He encouraged me to drink more grape Gatorade before I slinked into bed. He sat at the edge of the bed and said, "You are going to be okay. You are so strong, Nicole. Be patient and breathe." He pressed a warm washcloth to my forehead. I inhaled and exhaled and focused on breathing. I don't know how many breaths I took, but finally the Tylenol kicked in and I fell asleep.

Saturday, I met my friend Brittney for coffee. I was elated to see her because she had beautiful and kind energy. She was one of the coordinators of the benefit and I was able to thank her in person for all her hard work. We were also partners in the business Rochester Health and Fitness. This blog was a hub for all things healthy in the southeastern Minnesota area (unfortunately this took a backburner during my illness, and we never got it going again). We talked and talked and talked. Three hours had gone by and I realized I hadn't had any water or snacks. As we bid each other farewell I went home and made lunch. It was nearing 3 p.m. and I was hungry. I made a piece of toast with two scrambled eggs and half an avocado. I took one bite of the toast and thought I swallowed a razor blade. The back of my throat hurt so bad I could barely finish the food. I brewed hot tea to sip on. With each swallow it felt like thumb tacks were piercing the back of my throat. Later that evening, I heated a can of cream of chicken soup and went to bed hoping it wasn't strep throat or a terrible cold.

Nicole L. Czarnomski

The next morning, I woke to scads of cold sores in my mouth. They were on my tongue, under my tongue, on the left, on the right, and in the corner of my mouth and throat. These were no ordinary cold sores, these felt like they were on steroids which I guess could be true with all the steroids pumping through me.

My diet consisted of soft and mushy items. I drank smoothies and ate soup for days. I phoned the doctor on-call one night, and he recommended Tylenol for the pain. He encouraged me to finish off any leftover pain killers from previous surgeries. He recommended a saltwater bath for my mouth. I concocted a warm salty solution and swished it around my mouth hoping for relief. I hated Popsicles for being slackers.

On Monday morning, the sores were still camping inside my mouth despite the multiple saltwater gargles and Tylenol. My throat was on the mend, but my tongue felt like I dropped it in a blender and pressed the pulse button. This was the first time on the journey I felt completely defeated. I was hopeless and losing faith in my strength. I wanted to call my doctor and give him a big F.U. I hated Rachel for selling me chemo. I felt like a sucker for believing her. I wanted to return the chemo, all of it. I wanted to quit my new career: taking care of my feeble body. I hated this job more than anything in my life. I wanted a different challenge. I didn't want to be the girl with breast cancer anymore. I no longer believed all the stupid hashtags I added to my Facebook posts. #Warrior. #FightingTheGoodFight. What kind of crap was that? I was no warrior. I was weak and pathetic, and I wanted out.

I decided to do something about it. Standing on my yoga mat, I reached toward the sky inhaling and performed a swan dive exhaling all the air from my lungs. I completed multiple sun salutations as I followed along with the video. Once I finished, I laced up my sneakers, put on a light jacket and stocking cap to keep my bald head warm. The air was cold, and the sky was almost dark at 4:45 p.m. I chanted during the walk, "I am healthy and cancer-free. I am healthy and cancer-free." When I entered the house after my walk, I wasn't the same person. A transformation occurred, and I was stronger than when I walked out that door. The word spiritual badass was tattooed in my mind. Twenty minutes of beginner Vinyasa yoga on YouTube and a brisk, hour long walk saved me that day.

Later that evening, after a shower, Adlai blasted Lady Gaga's hit song Pokerface on our stereo system. "Muh, muh, muh, muh," I sang along and danced around the living room celebrating my renewed energy levels. Tylenol tamed the angry mouth sores only if I wasn't eating or drinking. I was happy again for a moment, and I forgot about the poison pulsing through my body.

After dancing around the living room, I took out my perfectly plump boobies with scars from armpit to sternum, flirted with my husband, and jumped in the sack. We rolled around and giggled like grade school kids. He gave me raspberries on my stomach which made us laugh even harder. And soon we settled into each other's arms. His patient hands helped prepare me for intimacy. He and my daisy downstairs melted into each other and the love I felt for him far exceeded any negative emotions chemo could ever give me. #FuckCancer.

# Psych!

Although I was still feeling weak, I was ready for my next chemo appointment. At least I thought I was. My dear friend Katie agreed to spend the day at the clinic with me as I went through my fourth and final round with the Red Devil. I was excited and worried. Round three brought me to my knees and I joked that I may be six feet under after round four. Only too late did I realize that wasn't funny.

The appointments started like any other appointment. I went and had my blood drawn which took all of 30 seconds. Then, I took Katie out to lunch at Newt's. I loved hanging out with her. She is one of the easiest people in the world to talk to and she is so down to earth. We bumped into Tami, another Fitness Friend, and she said her afternoon was open and she would stop by my chemo room later that afternoon.

After lunch, we went to the hat shop. I wanted a couple of new hats to keep me comfortable while indoors. Many of my hats were warm and cozy and great for outside, but not suitable for inside. We giggled as I tried on hats. I looked to Katie for her opinion and could tell by the look on her face when I put on a ridiculous hat. When she smiled, I knew it was a keeper, but when her grin turned to a grimace, I knew the hat had to go. I tried on hats faster than a magician juggling fire sticks, and we cackled like a couple of hens.

One of the hats had two long tails. Really long tails. The tails reached all the way to my buttocks. We giggled again at how ridiculous I looked. Without missing a beat, I said, "Bald girl problem number 43, finding the perfect hat for a girl with chemo."

I finally settled on a few lightweight hats and we were on our way to the next appointment. I checked in and Katie found a table where we could spread out and color. I brought my Swear Word coloring book courtesy of the Fitness Friends and Desert Dreams courtesy of my mom's best friend, Barb, who lives in the southwest. I sat down with Katie and pulled out the books and markers. Before I had a chance to select my coloring page, she was already coloring her page from the Swear Word book. My pager vibrated and beeped.

The nurse's assistant took my temperature and weight and led me back to a room. I was 40 minutes early to my appointment with the oncologist and I was excited at the thought of getting out of there early. The last two times I have waited more than 45 minutes to speak with him. The nurse's assistant took my blood pressure which presented problem number one. My blood pressure was 81 over 55. I looked at her and she looked at me. I put on my best no big deal face, but she said, "We should try again." I tried to comfort her.

I said, "Oh it's usually pretty low. My blood pressure hovers around 96 over 60 or 65. I am sure everything is fine." And I wasn't lying, my blood pressure was usually low, but I was actually a little scared when it registered 81 over 55.

She took it again and it registered 79 over 55. At that point, my gut was telling me this wasn't good. In fact, this was very bad. I suffered from dizzy spells a lot after round three of chemo and wondered if it was because my blood pressure was too low. I had been drinking Gatorade, but it was clearly slacking on the job.

A nurse came in and began asking me lots of questions. I wondered if it was because of my blood pressure. She was probably super excited to meet someone who had such low blood pressure and was still functioning. We went through everything. From having a dry daisy downstairs to dizzy spells. We talked about the rash across my chest, the horrible and multiple mouth sores, fatigue, severe nausea, the terrible migraines, specifically the one that left me whimpering in the shower, and finally the two visits from Fancy Pants (my menstrual period), yes, two visits in about three weeks. I started to feel

Nicole L. Czarnomski

uncomfortable talking about all the side effects and wondered how in the hell I was going to make it through round number four with the Red Devil.

At 3:30 p.m., an hour and 10 minutes past my regular scheduled time with my oncologist, and five minutes from my chemo appointment, I was still waiting. My oncologist arrived with another doctor. He introduced me to the gentleman, a pathologist who worked on human epidermal growth factor receptor 2, or HER2.

"Wait, what? Do I have something else wrong with me?" I asked.

"No, no. Everything is fine. The pathologist is shadowing me today to see what it's like to visit with patients. Everything is okay," he said. I was relieved to know there was nothing wrong with me, until he postponed round four.

"Postponed! Why?" I asked and right on cue, the tears arrived. There was nothing holding those tears inside of me, and nothing holding in the snot that was now running into my mouth. I grabbed a tissue from the box my oncologist sat in front of me.

This was frustrating and didn't make any sense. My body was wrecked for almost two weeks. It would seem logical to want to celebrate a little reprieve, but not me. I was ready to duke it out with the Red Devil for the last time. I had friends out in the waiting room that had come to celebrate my last aggressive chemo treatment. My friend Katie spent the entire day with me, I'll be damned if I was going to walk out there and tell her it was postponed.

"Let's take my blood pressure one more time! Please!" I begged.

"Nicole, it's more than having low blood pressure, although this tells me you are probably dehydrated," he said.

"No, that's just not possible. I have had 1500 ml of water today. I drank three cups of water since I arrived in this very office. Take it again. Please, let's just take my blood pressure one more time," I pleaded with him. I was acting like a child.

"Nicole, this is about the side effects your body has endured over the last couple of weeks. You need to let us know when things are this bad. We told you chemo wasn't going to be a walk in the park, but we also said you shouldn't be miserable," he said.

I needed to step away from the situation. Tears were still falling down my face and my head was hot. I ripped off my hat and set it next to me. I wiped my eyes and looked at my tissue; there was black all over it. "Look at this." I held out my tissue to show him. "You ruined my make-up for today. Do I have black circles under my eyes?" I asked in him in a huff.

"No, no. There are no black circles under your eyes," he said. "There's the humor we both know and appreciate," he smiled.

I felt slightly better knowing I wasn't sitting there in a puddle of make-up, so I put my hat back on and pulled myself together.

"Why are you so upset that you are missing this round of chemo?" He asked.

"My friends are here. I am so excited to get this last round over with so I can move on," I said.

My oncologist said, "Sometimes this happens. Sometimes we postpone treatment because we are concerned about our patient's health." And then he pulled the hospital card. "If I give you this round of chemo today, it's likely you will end up in the hospital with an IV full of antibiotics and saline because of an infection and dehydration," he said.

Damn. How could I argue with that? I hated hospitals as much as I hated needles and barfing. I wondered if there was a phobia of hospitals. I should google that when I get home.

"Fine. Can we reschedule for Monday?" I asked.

"How about next Friday?" he asked.

"Friday! Seriously? A whole week?" I freaked again. This cancer thing was really pissing me off today. Just yesterday I had stopped into my place of employment to drop off a few thank you cards and to say hello. I was feeling better, still a little light-headed, but I wanted to keep that quiet. I was so excited to see everyone. I received hugs and a warm welcome. I wanted to go back to work. I wanted normalcy. I wanted my damn life back. Going back to work felt like that was the closest thing to normalcy as I could get.

"Maybe, we could postpone the next chemo treatment until Wednesday or Thursday?" he said.

"Maybe, we could postpone and reschedule for Monday," I said again.

"Let's look at Tuesday or Wednesday," he said. I knew even though he said Tuesday or Wednesday, he meant Thursday or Friday. He was serious about the hospital and I knew it. He had probably seen it happen time and again and didn't want to see me suffer any more than I had in the last couple of weeks. In a way, I appreciated him, and in a way, I just wanted to throat punch him.

I walked out of the office and started to cry again. When I walked out to the waiting area, my friend Brittney, Katie, Tami, and

Sarah were coloring. They were having so much fun and here I was feeling sorry for myself.

"Oh my God, what's wrong?" asked Katie.

"They are postponing my chemo treatment until next week," I said. I explained the situation and they all looked at me with loving and supportive eyes. It was hug time. Katie whispered, "A hug is more meaningful if you hold it for 20 seconds." We stood there hugging while I cried and made sure my hug was 20 seconds long. I hugged each one of the other girls and felt better knowing I had a good support team.

I apologized to everyone for trying to hang out with me for no reason. They were awestruck by the comment. Sarah said, "We're here to support you." We sat there talking for several minutes after my appointment. Soon the waiting area cleared out and there was no one left. It was after five, so we all parted ways.

When we arrived back at my house, I invited Katie in for a beer. She sure deserved one after spending all day at the clinic with me and then putting up with me as I cried on her shoulder because they weren't going to inject me with poison. Adlai, Katie, and I stood around talking and indulging in pudding shots courtesy of my friend Sarah. I had a stash of about 18 left and guess what? We finished them all, including me. Yes, they do have alcohol, but trace amounts, so I figured it wouldn't matter. And it didn't.

The few days after the dreaded postponement were much better. I had an appetite; the dizzy spells and headaches went away. The mouth sores were gone, and my rash was healing. Each day I started feeling better and better. Truthfully, I was glad my oncologist postponed my chemo date, but don't tell him.

I received the call Tuesday morning, the Tuesday morning prior to my Wednesday treatment. It was the clinic asking to reschedule my chemo appointment from Wednesday until Thursday. "I'm sorry, we just don't have room in our schedule on Wednesday," the receptionist said. Damn, he got me from afar and didn't have to deal with me blubbering in his office again. Well played doctor man, well played.

I am so glad my oncologist made me wait a week before administering the last dose of the Red Devil. During that week, I was able to enjoy life again. And by the time my fourth round of chemo rolled around my blood pressure was back up to normal again, 95 over 66. Perfect.

Adlai took the day off to come with me. My appointment was at 8 a.m. and I was glad to get it out of the way. When the nurse arrived to put the IV in, I said, "I bet you are a pro at putting in IVs, right?"

He paused for what seemed like forever and finally said, "Well, I just finished with orientation, so I hope I get the first try." We laughed, but inside a little part of me was about to lose it. We talked a bit about needles, and I asked if everyone who came in was braver than me about them.

He said, "Ya know, it's kind of funny, you would think the more needles that were injected in someone would make them blasé about the whole experience, but it doesn't. No one really gets used to the idea of having a needle poked in their arm." It was somewhat of a relief to know that it wasn't just me who feared the almighty needle.

The IV was in place and the Red Devil was ready to dance. I received good news when the nurse wielding the Red Devil arrived. My oncologist had changed the dosage. He reduced the amount of Cytoxan and Adriamycin, or the Red Devil, by twenty percent. I was elated and terrified all at once. I was so excited the dosage was reduced because I was hopeful there would be less suffering, but terrified because of how brutal the last treatment was on my body. I wondered if there was any permanent damage to vital organs, my heart specifically. I remembered him telling me how bad this treatment was on a person's heart. It made me wonder about exercising again. Is cardio going to be too difficult for me when this is all over? Would I be able to lace up my tennis shoes and run the streets of my small town again?

Once the nurse started administering the Red Devil, I could feel the burning sensation run through my veins. I don't know why I was noticing this so intensely for the first time. Was the nurse pushing it through too quickly? Was my body simply tired of the torture? I mentioned something to the nurse, and she said she would push less poison through and let more of the saline drip into my system. Well she didn't call it poison, but I was sure she was thinking that.

My friend Brittney came to hang out with me for the last round as well. Adlai, Britt and I chatted throughout my last round until it was time to go. I was finished. Now, I had to wait for the side effects to hit. As we walked to the car, I kept thinking about how the steroids would keep me up at night. I thought about the nausea, headaches, dizzy spells, mouth sores, and all things I would need to brace myself for.

The rest of the day was uneventful. I spent a lot of time sitting and snoozing on the sofa. The steroids hadn't yet taken effect. The days that followed were uneventful as well. I had some difficulty sleeping the first few nights, but the Ativan helped with that. I was at least able to get a good six to seven hours in.

My last treatment went very well. I experienced some nausea, but the pills helped with that. I had a few mouth sores start, but a saltwater rinse seemed to help. They weren't as painful. I had a good appetite and was able to eat things that weren't bland and mushy.

This was my last dance with the Red Devil, and it turned out I was the one taking the lead this time.

The following week was Thanksgiving. Each year, Turkey Day was a quiet celebration for Adlai and I. Adlai's parents are in Florida and mine are in Missouri, so we opt to celebrate with our own turkey dinner and a hike. We've hiked through the hills and valleys of Whitewater State Park many times, and one year we ventured to Red Wing.

This year, one of the fitness studios where I worked pre-cancer hosted a Turkey Trot and dedicated it to me. Once again, I was astounded at the kindness and generosity of the human spirit. While I taught a class or two over the past couple of years at this location, I didn't know a lot of the people in the community but that didn't stop them from making generous donations towards my battle with cancer. The fire department even kicked in a substantial donation to assist with my medical bills.

The sun beamed on that Thursday, shining bright on all the good people in the community. Though the temperatures were low forties, the love surrounding me kept me warm and toasty for the 5K. Many people ran, but Adlai and another coach walked with me.

At the end of the walk/run, the owners of the studio presented me with all the donations. I walked to the front of the crowd with my head held high, finally proud of the woman that so many people loved and cared for. When I reached the front of the crowd, tears stung my eyes. I looked out at the crowd and stammered through a thank you speech that I felt would never be enough to express my gratitude. It seemed like every corner I turned these days, I found something beautiful waiting for me, something precious to make life worth living.

# Back in the Saddle

In late November 2017, I returned to work after a four-month absence. I bounced between fear and joy. Did the cancer or the chemo take away my ability to function in a work setting? How would I manage the fatigue? Would I catch all the germs floating around and get an infection? Despite my anxieties, Adlai and I needed my steady paycheck, and I needed the health insurance. I had to make it work. I now had multiple full-time jobs: working for my employer, managing self-care, and fighting cancer.

When I arrived back at the office, I received a warm welcome from everyone around me. I worked in marketing at a senior living community. My co-workers welcomed me, and the residents flooded me with hugs. Everyone had been so supportive through each phase of my journey. Thoughtful cards and prayers arrived in my mailbox and on my Facebook feed from so many wonderful people. One resident even referred to me as her Survivor Sister as she too battled breast cancer and beat it. (Though I hadn't beaten cancer yet, there was no doubt I would conquer this grueling mission.)

I loved my job at the senior living community, but it was challenging for me mentally and physically. The main reason I loved my job was because of the residents. I worked with grandmas and grandpas all day long. The other reason I liked this job was because of the hectic pace, but fighting cancer made the constant interruptions and daily tasks brutal. There were so many past due phone calls to make. We kept information in a database of everyone we worked with and tried to touch base with them every few months or so. You can imagine the backlog of calls I had from being away for so long. I had to give tours to people almost daily which meant constant interaction with the public, and I had no idea what germs people were bringing through the doors.

The first week back, my to-do list sucked the energy from my frail body; the four-month backlog forced me to take things in small bites and focus on gratitude. Whenever I had an overwhelming moment, I would whisper to the Universe, "I am grateful my employer is so caring and flexible." Each day I strived to do my best and hoped it was enough.

Doctor's appointments and weekly chemo treatments competed for my time with daily work tasks. I met with my nurse educator the first week back at the office, so she could sell me on Paclitaxel (Taxol). No time to kick the tires this time; my oncologist scheduled my first Taxol treatment for Friday. If you can imagine, Taxol frightened me more than the Red Devil because it could cause neuropathy. This meant possibly losing feeling in my fingers, hands, toes, and feet, affecting my ability to hold pens or pencils, button a shirt, or put on earrings and necklaces. Rachel told me to keep my fingernails and toenails trimmed because the nail beds would likely become irritated and painful. In some cases, the nail could separate from the nail bed and fall off.

Taxol was an allergen, so my body would be pumped full of Benadryl prior to the treatment. If the medication escaped from the vein it could cause tissue damage. She went on to talk about the severity of allergic reactions. Fear set up camp in my mind, I felt like someone grabbed my throat and squeezed slowly the same way a boa constrictor wrapped around its prey squeezing until the last breath evaporated.

"If you experience pain, notice redness, or swelling at the IV site while you are receiving Taxol, alert your nurse immediately," she said. "It will be beneficial to have someone drive you to treatments because of the side effects of the Benadryl. In some cases, you may be too tired to function behind the wheel of an automobile."

After she left, I didn't want to purchase the new chemo drug, but this was my only option unless I refused treatments which seemed ignorant. I sat fidgeting in the doctor's office and trembled when my oncologist entered the room with his customary smile and jovial hello. This was my first visit subsequent to him postponing my last round with the Red Devil. I swallowed my pride and admitted to him that I was being stubborn when he cancelled my last treatment. I thanked him for postponing my treatment, and for reducing the dosage. "I breezed through my last two weeks with very few side effects," I said.

He laughed and asked, "You knew you weren't going to win the fight with me, right?"

"Yes, but I wasn't going down without a fight. I just wanted it to be over. The Red Devil was challenging," I said.

"I know," he said. "That's why we delayed it. I am glad you found more comfort during the last round." Comfort seemed like an odd description, but true, nonetheless.

He pushed his dark framed glasses up on his nose with his middle finger and started talking about Taxol. His facial expression conveyed the serious nature of the drug.

"It's very important for you to communicate with us about Taxol. We don't want nerve damage." He told me that many people in the past have tried to 'power through it' and ended up with permanent nerve damage. "Taxol's side effects are irreversible, so if you lose feeling in your hands, feet, arms, or legs for more than a couple of days, you must let us know. If you develop neuropathy, we will postpone treatment, or towards the end of treatment, we may cut it short." My attitude lightened when he said cut my treatments short. At first it sounded awesome, but the more I thought about it, the more scared I became. I realized Taxol's power; it had the upper hand.

I left the office terrified but was determined to communicate this time; stubborn was not an option. I blasted through many terrifying challenges in this journey, but this part felt more intimidating. The idea of irreversible side effects was alarming. I had made it through surgery, and though, underneath my clothing, my breasts would never look the same, on the outside people were none the wiser. I survived the Red Devil, and the side effects would soon disappear, but Taxol was a whole different beast. The idea of neuropathy left me chugging uphill on an emotional roller coaster.

I waited for my first round of Taxol while anxiety built up. During the first leg of treatment, the nurse pumped Benadryl into my system through an IV. It burned and tingled in the crook of my arm. Steroids weaved their way into my system to combat fatigue, followed by Pepcid to help with acid reflux and nausea. Physically, my body was prepared for Taxol. Mentally, terror ransacked the cells in my brain.

The poisonous fluid entered my body as the nurse stood close and watched over me. The tension was palpable, her expression serious, unrelenting. I waited for the injection site to burn or turn red. It felt like I was standing in water up to my nose, waiting for it to rise just one more inch. Soon, I would be fully emerged and unable to breathe. Minutes passed, but nothing happened. I observed as the nurse checked the watch on her left wrist. I put my chair in a reclined position and pushed the button on the remote for a light massage. I shut my eyes and started breathing with intention. Inhale. Exhale. Inhale. Exhale. After five painstaking minutes, the nurse smiled and said I was in the clear, no allergic reaction. I sighed loud enough for the neighboring room to hear me, but no one commented. The only side effect plaguing me at this moment was caused by the Benadryl. I yearned to fall asleep, but the Benadryl didn't have enough power to send me into the REM state. I sat in my chair repeating in mind, I am strong, healthy, and cancer-free. The treatment was over in about an hour, and I had the weekend to recover before going back to work on Monday.

I worked 32 hours a week during Taxol treatments. While my doctor didn't recommend it, I made it work. With Taxol, I couldn't be given Neulasta, the man-made form of protein that stimulates the growth of white blood cells, because my treatments were weekly, and the Taxol would kill off all the proteins. This meant my white blood cell count could plummet, making me more susceptible to infections.

One afternoon at work, I started having chest pains. Was it the pressures at work or Taxol? Was I having a heart attack? Or a panic attack? Should I take Ativan, or baby aspirin? The pains were minor, but unsettling.

My four-month vacation from work (if you could call it that) made it easier to find time for self-care. I had discovered wellness on a whole new level. I engaged in walking, doing yoga, and meditating. Now, because there was so much to accomplish at work during the day, I left the office exhausted with little time and energy to care for my mental, physical, and emotional health. The days were tiresome. If I did have an ounce of energy left after work, the cold, dark days of November and December left me weary and unmotivated.

I tried to exercise at work in our health club over my lunch hour but there usually wasn't time. I put so much pressure on myself to keep up and be a part of the team again. The people I worked with had to pick up the slack while I was out, and I was grateful. But now, it felt like I needed to make up for lost time and take the burden off them.

Mentally, exhaustion captured the blue ribbon as I struggled to keep up. Sadly, I looked forward to my treatment days because I was able to go home and sleep. My thoughts grew dark while chemo and cancer sent death threats to me. These thoughts stuck inside my brain like a spoon of peanut butter on the roof of my mouth. I despised the thought of not traveling to all the places I wanted to go and accomplishing all the dreams I had tucked away in my mind. What if all the work I had done in my four-month absence was for naught, the surgery, the physical therapy, the first several rounds of chemo, was it a waste of time, money, and effort? Was I going to die? My heart ached, I was distressed; I had to make time for self-care and exercise, or the darkness in my mind would win the battle.

When I arrived home after work each evening, I wrapped myself in a coat and hat, and I walked outside in the dark reminiscing about the mostly positive attitude I had while away from work. In the four months I spent with myself, I fell in love with the new me. Over the years, I had said so many hurtful things to myself, and I wondered if I had given myself cancer. Those four months helped me realize the importance of the thoughts in my brain. And those thoughts must be positive. I was enough. Life was as fragile as a soap bubble glistening in the sunlight.

Each day, I pushed myself to find one thing to be grateful for and held that thought in my mind when I felt stressed. My self-talk changed, and I repeated, I am strong, resilient, and I'm a beautiful person. It was important to remember that wellness lies within, it was a matter of tapping into it every moment. Being grateful for one thing led to two things, and then three, and four. My grateful attitude bloomed every day. I regained the self-care routines I needed, and I confidently pushed through each day. At that point, I also realized how easy it was to revert to the old me, the critical me. It was so easy to berate myself and choose harmful words over healthy ones. Just like I couldn't see the cancer that was hurting me, I hadn't seen how powerful negative thoughts were either. Fighting cancer was just as hard as fighting off negative thoughts.

Nicole L. Czarnomski

I breezed through round one and two of Taxol, but round three was cancelled because my white blood cell count was too low. Unless I missed multiple treatments, I would skip round three and it would be forgotten like a phone number in the age of cell phones. I was frustrated; I made the 30-minute drive for nothing but another needle stick. Since my right arm was out of commission, thanks to cancer spreading to my lymph nodes, my left arm caught the brunt of every needle and was basically a fleshy pin cushion. Some of my poor veins looked bruised under the skin, and I wondered if they would collapse. In hindsight, I should have chosen the port.

The nurse sent me home with a mask and said to wear it and stay healthy. I was typically a rule follower when it came to medical issues, but that day I became a rebel. Angry and fed up with cancer, needles, and chemo, I left the clinic with my mask stowed in my purse instead of on my face.

My friend Carrie, who brought me to that appointment, remained patient and kind. She said she didn't mind driving me to my cancelled appointment. She reminded me that they were just skipping this treatment. "You should be happy you don't have to have treatment today," she said with a smile, and then took me to the mall, so I could do my Christmas shopping. I shopped without my mask and went home and slept. I managed to stay healthy even sans mask. Going rogue felt good for a change.

Round four scared the shit out of me. In the middle of my treatment, I had my chair reclined so far back I was almost all horizontal. I lay cloaked in a warm, white blanket, my body full of Benadryl and Taxol. Each breath shallow, my chest felt like my rib cage was in a vice. After about five minutes, I pressed my call button and mentioned my symptoms to one nurse. She shut off the Taxol and suddenly five more nurses were in my room. They hovered over me like members of a football team huddled together before a last-minute play. One nurse stopped the Taxol drip, and checked my oxygen levels. They took my blood pressure. My temperature. All my vitals were good. They kept asking me how I felt. I said with a breathy voice, "I just can't breathe very well. My chest…tight." With each minute that passed, the nurses looked more concerned. There was nothing wrong with me, but everything was wrong with me. Their helpless faces worried me. Should I shut my eyes and let go? Was this my final moment? Stranded in a chemo ward with caring nurses who were all strangers to me? They paged my oncologist. While waiting to hear from him, one of the nurses set a timer and stayed in my room watching over me like a mama bear.

I put my chair back up to the seated position. Within five minutes, the vice grip on my chest released, and I took a deep breath like someone swimming up from the bottom of a lake after holding their breath 20 seconds too long. The nurse continued to monitor me while I sat there. "I feel better," I said. "I can breathe again." She turned on the Taxol, and soon my treatment commenced. Soon, the only side effect that plagued my body was from the Benadryl. I felt like I was sleeping one off in the drunk tank, not that I would know anything about the drunk tank.

I wanted to cry. I was embarrassed and anxious. Why did that happen? Why was my chest so tight? Was there a correlation to the chest pains I had had last week? My eyelids were tired from the weight of the tears. I wanted to cry, but I didn't want to alarm the nurses again. My chest started to tighten as I held back tears. Stop it! I said to myself. I was tough, right? The 'warrior' as my friends called me, slowly returned. I repeated my mantra, "I am strong, healthy, resilient, and cancer-free."

Inhale...exhale...

My friend Sarah arrived. She was my strength that day, and knowing Sarah, belly laughs were around the corner. I wanted to be strong for her. I wanted her to know that I was still rocking this cancer/chemo thing. I wasn't going down without a fight. All my friends and family reminded me at the beginning of this journey that I possessed an extraordinary amount of strength. Now, they wondered how I managed to walk down this difficult path and maintain a sense of humor and exhibit so much grace. I secretly lied to all of them. Some days, I was far from a warrior, no strength or grace in sight. I pasted a smile across my face shrouding any evidence of fear.

With Sarah in my room, my negative thought patterns ceased. Gratitude filled my heart and soul. She stayed and chatted for a while and left me in high spirits. No more tears from this strong and ferocious warrior everyone talked about. I hid the fake smile in my back pocket for another day.

The following day, Adlai and I took our first long road trip since my cancer diagnosis. My oncologist had cleared me for a trip outside of the state, so we would be celebrating Christmas with my family in Missouri several hours away. This Christmas felt more special than any other. I had endured so much over the past several months, and I was still able to live life with gratitude and a smile most days.

Adlai and I had made two homemade decorative signs made from pallet wood for Angie and MeMe. Popps and my brother were getting Green Hornet fishing poles, ones from "Grumpy Old Men", a favorite movie of theirs. We had purchased my grandma a nightlight and my niece a gift card to Victoria's Secret. I loved giving gifts.

Though our budget was smaller that year because I was off work for so long, we managed to find a few things for everyone, and I couldn't wait for all of them to open their presents. I cherished my time with them, and I was so grateful for their support and unconditional love.

My mom stuffed us full of delicious meals every day, we laughed, played cards, and on Christmas Eve drove around Binder Lake to watch the holiday light show. Each night, I fell asleep grateful to spend another Christmas with the people I loved the most, grateful for my surgeons, my chemo team, and all the people around me who bathed me with love and support.

After the holidays, I was thrust back into the hectic pace at work. While I had thought a lot about my lifestyle during the four-month hiatus from work, I learned the importance of using my mind to truly manifest what I wanted. I discovered that manifesting desires was a more delicate and profound process than I originally thought. "Thoughts become things, choose the good ones," stated Jack Dooley, author of Notes from the Universe website. I had been receiving "messages" from the Universe for many years. They pop up in my inbox each day with a positive message and are designed to help me see my dreams becoming a reality. I have enjoyed these messages for many years and believed I understood the importance of each of them.

As my journey continued, I pondered the past and saw that I hadn't taken the time to appreciate everything I built along the way. It was incredibly easy to let stress, worry, and fear penetrate the forefront of my mind. All my life, I chased goals as if they were items on a grocery list. I checked them off and moved on. I never slowed down to be grateful for the items piling up in my grocery cart, never celebrating small victories. My Fitness Friends taught me to celebrate each new challenge and every victory along the way no matter how large or small.

My cancer diagnosis was my cue to slow down and listen. I stopped teaching fitness classes, I stopped freelancing for local publications so I could focus on fighting and healing. Though disappointing to let go, they were jobs, not the essence of who I was. I could still exercise, albeit on a whole new level while battling cancer, and I could write in my journal, satisfying the desire to write. When I found myself sandwiched between fear and love, my friend Beverly helped give me a voice to the emotions that at times were too terrifying to put in my journal. Writing made the journey, the cancer more real, but it was cathartic. She urged me to continue writing about my journey because one day I would be able to share my story with others.

One cold Sunday in January of 2018, Beverly and I discussed interesting information we learned from a writer's workshop we attended a little over a year ago, a mere five months before my diagnosis. Putting pen to paper was scarce that weekend, but I had the opportunity to take the Passion Test and meet a group of women who all wanted to have a voice, to be more than a job title, and to accept challenges so they could face their fears. These women were all looking to better their lives.

At this workshop in February of 2017, I learned about the Passion Test, created by Janet Bray Attwood and Chris Attwood. It helped me discover my passions and how to breathe life into them. The workshop helped me identify my top 10 passions and from there, my top five passions. My top five were: to be healthy, have a loving relationship with my husband, surround myself with kind and loving people, write a book, and travel.

I wrote these desires on a notecard and left the workshop feeling empowered. But I fell short with these desires soon after the workshop. As Beverly and I revisited the items from my Passion Test, we wrestled with these ideals, and she helped me become more specific in hopes of rekindling the ideas for my perfect life.

After the phone conversation, I sat with the idea of good health in my head while I created a journal entry for this passion. I used positive desires and used them as a mantra. I spoke these desires as if I already had them in my life. My mantra was, I am cancer-free, healthy, slim, yet strong. I practice yoga at least four times a week. I take daily walks. I eat healthy foods for fuel.

My next passion was to be in a loving relationship with my husband. My mantra was, I love and support my husband. I am grateful for his support through my cancer journey. We have a symbiotic relationship and cater to our sexual desires. We enjoy spending time together even doing the mundane chores in life like grocery shopping. We make time to travel and try new things.

My third passion was to be surrounded by kind and loving people. My goal is to love people through good and bad times, show my friends and family support like they have shown me through the difficult journey and beyond.

My fourth passion was to write a book, but at the time of the workshop, I had no idea what to write about. I wrote down ideas on note cards, but nothing felt right until I was diagnosed with cancer. I knew then, this was my story to tell. My book inspires people to overcome adversity through self-care, positive self-talk, and a positive attitude. I want to help people find humor in ugly, uncomfortable situations in life and live each day to the fullest because we never know when our last breath will be taken.

My fifth passion was travel. I travel to explore and learn. I travel to promote my book and teach people to write for healing.

These passions became obsessions. I wanted these passions in my life, so I tried to focus on them every day. I returned to the page time and again and used the time to express gratitude, to remember and feel fear that surfaced especially on the days that I watched poison being injected into my body. The journal was a safe space, and I believe these pages saved my life and taught me to be laser-focused on the good surrounding me.

So much had changed at work and for me personally while completing my Taxol treatments. I felt almost like a stranger observing from the outside. It was difficult to believe that this was my life. I was thin and bald everywhere. There wasn't one hair on my entire body. I wore a hat every day, and I had to draw eyebrows on because I felt I looked sick without them. Eyelashes were also a thing of the past. I looked in the mirror every morning and forced myself to smile at the stranger in front of me.

I no longer exercised with the intensity that I was used to. In fact, I never broke a sweat. Instead I walked when I had the energy and completed 10, 20, and 30-minute yoga videos.

Sometimes I would literally ask myself, "Who is this girl?" I often wondered if this was the new me or if I would return to the girl I was one year ago. It didn't matter, I needed to focus on healing.

At work, corporate searched for candidates to fill the open positions. My colleagues and I wondered who would be joining our team and how new hires would fit in. Fortunately, we had an excellent interim executive director who had been with the company for many years. He kept the team on the right path. He was an excellent leader and kept the work atmosphere incredibly positive.

Meanwhile, I tried to focus on each aspect of my job, though some days were challenging. The fatigue was overwhelming, and I wanted to be focused on me and only me. I wanted that time to be selfish again. Although, I was working 32 hours a week, it felt like 50. I fought to stay positive and healthy. By the time I returned home each night, fatigue often won the battle, and I fell asleep on the sofa longing for the energy I had pre-chemo. My body was robotic. Rise, work, sleep, repeat.

It was time for my next Taxol treatment. Adlai took off work to drive me to my appointment. I was feeling good and had a healthy appetite, so we decided to go to lunch together. We chose to eat at Hy-Vee because of the variety and simplicity of items on the menu. As we pulled into the parking lot, I noticed it right away. The Weiner Mobile was parked in front of the grocery store. With wide eyes and brows arched, I exclaimed, "Oh WOW!"

Adlai pulled Ginger, my red RAV-4, into the snow-packed parking spot. It was a brisk walk from the car through the sub-zero temperatures. It had been frigid for days, the kind of cold that seeps into the seams of your coat, hat, and gloves, and makes your skin want to hibernate. The cold weather didn't stop us from posing in front of the Weiner Mobile for a picture, standing in front of the garish vehicle and giggling as we snapped photos of each other.

We sent the pictures to my parents for a chuckle as we laughed and cracked jokes about wieners. "Did you see the license plate?" I asked Adlai.

"No, what did it say?" he asked.

"W. I. E.N.R. Wiener!" We laughed about wieners and wondered what it would be like to drive around in a wiener all day long. "Who applies for that job? Do they literally drive across the country visiting grocery stores selling wieners from the Wiener Mobile?" I asked. As we ate our lunch we continued to talk about wieners and our utter disgust for hotdogs. What a bizarre but gloriously normal morning.

After lunch, we drove to the clinic to see what was in store. Each day, and each treatment was always different.

I found myself sitting amongst other balding cancer patients and family members, waiting for my name to be called, waiting for another needle stick. As always, bloodwork was first to make sure my white blood cell count was strong enough for the next round of poison.

When my pager went off, I walked to my private room. I put my left arm up on the chair and waited for the needle. I thought I was becoming less anxious about needles. I inhaled a few deep breaths as the technician tied the orange rubber tourniquet and wiped my arm with a cold alcohol wipe. He waited a few seconds and plunged the needle into my bruised vein. Pain shot through my arm.

"Ouch! Why did that one hurt so much?" I asked.

"The needle may have hit a little scar tissue. It was difficult to insert," he said.

The next appointment was with my oncologist. He didn't keep us waiting long that day. He opened the doctor's office door with a wide toothy smile. I wondered if he ever walked into a room unhappy. I surmised that if he arrived in my room happy, it was because he didn't have any bad news for me. I briefly thought of what his sad or solemn face looked like and shoved that thought into my back pocket in hopes that I would never see it.

He reviewed my white blood cell counts with Adlai and me. Today they were almost normal. I had skipped the week prior because the counts were too low. My counts were 1.5 and normal is 1.7. This was the highest they had been since I started chemo. He said "This is very good, so we are going to treat you, but we are going to reduce the dosage by 20 percent. The goal is to keep you from skipping every third week." I was happy with that news.

When I got into my chemo room, the nurse complimented me on my hat. It was a crocheted olive-green hat with two brown buttons sewn slightly to the right and big furry puff ball on the top. One of the chemo nurses gave it to me. The nurses had all pitched in that year and purchased hats for patients instead of giving gifts to each other at Christmas.

My pre-chemo drugs were administered. My eyelids bobbed like a red and white fishing bobber as sleep knocked at my door. One by one, visitors arrived. My friend Denise stopped by on her break, and so did a Pink Ribbon Mentor. Conversation buzzed in my room, and I had a hard time focusing and tracking the conversation. My mouth was getting dry, my eyelids heavier. The Benadryl I was given made it tough to stay awake. I noticed my speech started to slur, and I realized I was back in the drunk tank.

I imagined the chemo ward, my drunk tank for that day, was probably like a drunk tank for Martha Stewart should she ever get caught three sheets to the wind and needing a place to stay. Her drunk tank would include a heated recliner with nurses (or really nice police officers) bringing in warm white blankets and pillows every hour to make her stay more comfortable. I imagined police officers bringing her goose liver pate, caviar, and sparkling water instead of Rice Krispie treats and apple juice. She could have her curtain pulled any time with lights dimmed for the ultimate in relaxation and healing. The frosted glass that separated the rooms, or cells if you will, kept her secret safe within the confines of an eight-foot by eight-foot chemo room or holding cell.

My visitors didn't stay long, probably because the Benadryl made me act drunk and sleepy. I closed my eyes and began to relax. I lay in my reclined, heated seat until someone new stopped by. "Hi, my name is Laura, and I'm with Caring Hands. Would you like a complementary hand massage?"

"Yes, please," I said wondering if she thought I was drunk too. She propped my right arm up on a pillow and sat down. She massaged the upper and lower side of my hand. The massage was wonderful. There was no talking, no worry of sounding drunk, just pure relaxation. I had no recollection of how long she spent with me.

When she was done, I asked if I could tip her. She put her hands up and waved her palms at me, "No, no. I am a volunteer," she said. "This service is free. I could get in a lot of trouble if I take your money." She smiled and went to find her next non-paying customer.

About thirty minutes after my hand massage, my bag of Taxol was empty, and the medicine was now floating around in my system ready to fight off any cancer that may still be in my system. The nurse unplugged the small catheter stuck in my arm, wrapped gauze around the entry, and I was released.

My next chemo appointment was in the afternoon again. I loved the afternoon appointments because it meant I got to sleep in. Adlai and I stopped at Chipotle for lunch. I was excited to eat at Chipotle; food was tasting better again. I was less nauseous with Taxol.

After lunch, we headed to the clinic. This was my routine. The new normal. It felt strange to find comfort in going for my treatments. My job was still to heal my broken body, and I was fighting like hell to do that. I told myself numerous times that this was a one-time thing, a one-night stand. One and done baby. I made it my duty to find time each day to continue repeating the mantra, I am cancer-free, I am healthy, I am resilient, and I am strong.

This routine made needles a little less scary each time. I went in and told the technician to find a different vein to draw from because the usual vein was tired. It was now a dark purplish hue that would have given grape Kool-Aid a run for its money. She smiled at me, "No problem." For a split second, anxiety shot through my body, and I wondered how well the other vein would handle the catheter. Did I screw myself? Was she going to have to wiggle around in my arm to stick another vein? Before I knew it, the needle was out, and she was wrapping the gauze around my arm. "Have a great day," she said as I walked out of the room.

I retrieved my second pager of the day, and minutes later, we walked into my room in the chemo ward, with every step I braced myself for another round of Taxol. When I arrived, my nurse came in. She was perky and chatty. I liked her. Her perky demeanor soon vanished, and she said my white blood cell count was too low for treatment. She said, "Last week you were at 1.5 and this week you dropped down to 1.0. Normally 1.0 was fine, but since you dropped so drastically from last week, I put a call into your oncologist, and I am waiting to hear back."

She went on to talk about low counts and hospitalization and wearing masks, and I tuned her out; after all, I knew the drill. She left my room to answer the page from my oncologist. Seconds later, she returned. "Okay, he wants to treat you, but we are going to continue with a dosage reduction."

"He reduced me 20 percent last week. Is he reducing another 20 percent?" I asked.

"No, no. It will be the same as last week. It's a 20 percent reduction from the original," she said. She left my room to go get my pre-meds ready.

I heard a rumble. I looked at my husband and he was smiling.

"Oh my God, you farted, didn't you?" I asked half laughing, half mortified.

"Maybe," He said with a smirk.

"Stop! The nurse is going to come back to fart air, and this will not be blamed on me!" I exclaimed.

He looked at me with wide eyes, "Shhhh!"

"What? Now you're getting shy. You don't want them to hear me say it, but it's okay for them to smell it?"

Damn. Chipotle! I thought to myself.

My nurse returned a few minutes later with pre-meds. She didn't make any faces, so I don't think she smelled anything. Many years ago, an unsuspecting woman at the grocery store walked right through one of Adlai's fart clouds. I felt bad for the poor lady as she scrunched her face, but not bad enough to stop laughing. It was one of those times when you laugh so hard it hurts.

The nurse administered the Benadryl, and I found myself in the sleepy, speech-slurring state. A Pink Ribbon Mentor came in while nurse Mishonda was in the room with me. The Pink Ribbon Mentor started talking to me about my surgery and chemo drugs and all the typical things that go along with breast cancer. Mishonda joined in the conversation and asked, "If there is one thing you could have known before all this started what would that be?"

I was stumped. I rummaged around in memories tucked away in my brain. It took a few seconds, but I finally responded. "I wish someone would have told me drains can remain securely in place for longer than 10 days. And remember to get another round of antibiotics if the drain remains in your body!" The Pink Ribbon Mentor and I swapped drain stories. And soon she left to tend to other patients.

Mishonda's question stayed with me after she left my room. I realized there was more I wish I would have known. Why wasn't I told birth control pills may cause breast cancer? Why wasn't I told that because I didn't have children, I was at a higher risk for breast cancer so I should have that mammogram at age 40 and do not wait until age 45?

I was shaken from contemplation by a rumbling vibration sound across the room. Yes, it was a fart. And then another.

"Oh my God, that is going to waft out into the common areas and everyone is going to think we are just fartin' it up in here. I swear I will tell the nurses it's you who is farting."

Adlai shushed me again like my words were worse than his farts, so I lay back in my fart-infested drunk tank.

"Go find me some apple juice and get some of that gas out of your system," I said.

He came back with some juice and farted again. I straight up lost it and erupted into laughter. The deep belly roll type of laugh. I couldn't help it anymore. Farts were funny. My stomach ached from the laughter; my head throbbed from the gigantic grin across my face. I had never laughed so hard at one of my chemo treatments, and I started to wonder if a nurse was going to come in and tell us to settle down. No one ever came. Maybe they knew laughter throughout the halls of a chemo ward was truly the best medicine.

When my treatment was completed, nurse Kathryn removed the catheter, and I walked out of my room. As I passed by nurse Mishonda she said, "Do you want a mask?"

I growled at her. Literally. Growled. Poor girl. An hour ago, I wanted to take her out to lunch and make her my new BFF because of her care and concern for my well-being, but now I just wanted to throat punch her.

She held up her hands and smiled. "Stop. Relax. Let me send a couple with you and you can decide. But I think it would be a good idea."

I took the two masks she gave me and shoved them into my purse. These masks were going to make me look like a sick person, and I refused to consider myself sick.

My chemo treatments were following a pattern. Two on, one off, two on, one off, so I was proactive this week. Thursday, the day before my treatment, I decided to have my blood levels checked. I felt worn down, I suffered from minor mouth sores, and the toenail on my right big toe was now almost entirely purple. I had showed it to the nurse last week and she said to keep monitoring it and watch for any puss.

I thought if I had my blood levels checked a day early, I wouldn't have to drive into town for nothing. I was surprised when the physician's assistant told me they were slightly low, but not too low to hold off treatment. Chemo number nine was on. She told me to continue swishing with saltwater for the mouth sores and watch the toe for oozing or puss.

The following day, I drove to my appointment alone. I discovered the Benadryl wore off by the time Taxol was flushed through my system so driving home would be fine. They prepped me for the drugs, and soon more of the poison was injected into my tired, purple vein. I was delighted when my friend Sarah arrived. It felt like months since we had seen each other. I was able to share my struggles to keep up at work and we talked about her most recent vacation to the Dominican Republic. She brought me Rice Krispie treats and reminded me that my punch card was almost full—my chemo punch card. And she was right. Three more to go and this chapter of my life would be complete. A cause for celebration.

My right big toe throbbed. The toenail was deep purple, so I purchased a new pair of shoes, so my toes had more room to breathe. These shoes were designed for either a three-year-old or an eighty-year-old. There was a Velcro strap across the top of a wide shoe base. The leather was engraved with a swirling floral pattern, and the soles were a cross between Dansko clogs and Crocs. Despite their ageist appearance the wide shoe base no longer smashed my toes inside, so it was worth it.

A few days after my chemo treatment with Sarah, my fingers went numb and stayed that way until my next treatment. That entire week I struggled to open Ziploc bags and pop tops on ginger ale and cat food lids. Was the neuropathy ever going to go away, or would I forever be asking my husband to help me open things.

When I arrived for chemo appointment number 10, I still had mouth sores, a tingling sensation in my fingers and toes and one disgusting looking toenail that was on the verge of falling off. One of the staff members was getting me prepped for chemo when the nurse arrived and said, "Don't get too comfortable. Your counts are the lowest they have been." She held up the paper exhibiting the low blood count reading so I could see it. It read .76. Despite the low counts, I was relieved to hear this news. I wanted to go home and rest. I didn't care if they tacked on another treatment because I had missed so many. My body was wearing out, and I was exhausted. How much more poison could my body handle? Walking to my car I thought about those masks in my purse and felt it might be a good idea to wear one this weekend if I go out in public. It was time to ignore my inner rebel.

The numbness in my fingers continued like a lingering, nasty cold. The sensation I felt in my fingers was what I imagined frostbite felt like. My fingertips tingled and any pressure applied felt like a lightning bolt ripping through my hands. The tips of my fingernails were turning a yellowish-brown and began to curl under with such force I thought they may fold in half. The edges of my nails were cracking. I had nail glue at my office and at home in case any nail finally broke. I wanted to avoid any more unwanted pain in my poor fingers. Gone were the days of beautifully manicured nails with sexy red or funky purple polish.

The week flew by, and it was time for my next treatment. I drove to town wondering if this was the end or if they were going to skip another appointment. I secretly hoped my white blood cell count was low again so they wouldn't treat me. I wanted to be done. I was prepared to walk in and tell my oncologist to please skip one more treatment. The neuropathy had reached scary levels. Opening sealed bags or jars was impossible now. At this point, I didn't care if he wanted to add an additional week to my treatments; I needed to rest before the next one.

I pulled into a spot on the third level repeating number three, number three, number three a trick I learned to use early on to remember my parking spot after treatments. I walked through the prickly cold air and took the stairs to the subway level. There was a piercing sensation in my fingertips as I clutched the purple railing. Walking into this building was like walking to work. Fighting cancer was my job, and this building was my office. I walked on the marble floor and took the elevator up 10 floors. I walked past the beautifully rendered wall of photographs telling the story of the founders of the hospital. I walked under the same intricate Chihuly glass sculptures suspended from the ceiling. The yellow, blue-green and clear glass twisted and contorted into organic shapes. The sculptures looked like they would be found in the far reaches of the ocean. I have always admired the work of Chihuly even before the days of cancer, chemo, and the renowned clinic that was helping me fight this disease.

The elevator was overcrowded giving me a hint of claustrophobia. The bleach blonde lady closest to the elevator door punched the number 10 for me. One by one everyone exited the elevator and finally stopped on level 10. I took a left off the elevator and was awed again by the bright sun shining through the floor to ceiling windows overlooking a historic old hotel.

I checked in for the blood draw and hoped my counts would be low. Pleading with the oncologist today sounded like way more effort than I had inside of me. I wanted to be cut loose. I wanted this chapter to end, and when it came down to it, I may have to be assertive and tell them to back off treatment.

The receptionist on floor number 10 smiled in my direction signaling me to approach the wood laminate desk. She asked my name and date of birth, and then passed a pager across the desk and told me to have a seat. My butt barely reached the chair when the pager went off. They were 10 minutes early for my appointment.

I sat in a large white chair, my feet barely touching the ground. I was acutely aware of my surroundings that day, anxious for the doctor to pull the plug on my treatment. I wanted that day to be the day the oncologist said, 'no more, you are done.' My left arm lay on the arm rest and I pushed my knitted sweater up to my bicep muscles which was not as muscular or defined as it once was. The nurse secured the orange rubber tourniquet around my arm and asked me to squeeze a small, white, wrapped piece of gauze. She pressed on both veins that surfaced and said ready for the poke. Most of the time, I turned my head away and tensed my entire body, but today, I felt the poke and looked at the syringe and needle sticking out from the crook of my elbow for the first time ever. The top container filled with blood. Three seconds went by and she pulled the needle from my arm and wrapped my elbow with gauze. I marveled at my strength and ambivalence towards this whole process. Three months ago, heck, a few weeks ago, I was clawing at my leg practically shredding my jeans because I looked at the stupid tourniquet. Now, I was literally facing my fear.

I had an hour to wait before my appointment with the oncologist, so I went to the subway level to get coffee. The storefronts in the subway were all dark, since it was so early. When I arrived at Caribou, there were 10 people standing and waiting for their order. I ordered a dark chocolate latte with almond milk and waited. One by one each person's name was called to pick up their drink. Within five minutes the warmth of the coffee cup spread through my cold, tingling hands.

I checked in again when I got back to the 10th floor. When my line of questioning at the front desk was completed, she handed me the pager and I walked to door C. There were several empty chairs, so I picked one away from people and filled out my questionnaire. It was the same one each week. Rate your pain level and describe where the pain is located. How is your overall outlook on life, blah, blah, blah? I answered all five questions letting them know about the severe neuropathy hoping they would read my pleading note and cancel my last two treatments without me having to say anything.

I set the paperwork aside and began staring at the black and white photographs on the opposite wall. I had seen these photos over and over and I always fixated on the same image. There was a man lying on the ground reaching to the sky, and there was another man doing a one-arm handstand on the first guy's extended arm. Both of their bodies were sculpted, sinewy. It made me think about the power of the mind and body. This feat could not occur if one of them lost concentration or skipped a day at the gym. The image was my life. I knew I would not win my battle with cancer unless I kept my mind sharp and filled with positive mantras as well as walking and stretching in yoga classes to keep my body healthy. I wondered if neuropathy was slowly dying inside of me while the positive mantras took over my mind, body, and soul.

My pager went off mid-thought. I gathered my belongings and went through the double doors. They were early with this appointment too. This could only mean one thing...they were going to cut me loose early because my counts were too low again.

I removed my shoes and stepped on the scale. I had shed 10 lbs since this all started and most of my pants were saggy and loose. The receptionist scribbled my height and weight on to a piece of paper and led me down the brightly lit hallway. The walls were a sterile shade of white. The door to each office had a secret code. There were rectangular plastic flags that would illuminate red or green lights to communicate with staff.

When I entered the office, I sat on the love seat that could easily fit four of me. The nurse took my blood pressure, which was the highest it had ever been since I started the Taxol treatment. This week it was 106 over 60. My pulse, which had been off the charts since I started chemo, was 90. As an athlete, the number disgusted me, and I was sure my seventh-grade track coach would be giving me suicide sprints as homework. "How disappointing," I could hear him say. Well, what the hell did he know about cancer anyway?

After the receptionist gathered the data needed for the doctor, she left the room and said the doctor would be available shortly. Rachel, the chemo salesperson, enter my room. Her grey tights were adorned with a bohemian print, and her black, gray, and white top matched. "Rachel, what a wonderful surprise, I am so happy to see you!" I exclaimed peering at her name badge secured with a brightly colored rhinestone clip. Her voice was pleasant, and she responded with the same sentiments.

"I hear you are having some trouble with neuropathy," she said.

"Yes," my eyes welled up for just a moment before the tears dissipated.

"Do you think the feeling will come back? I can't open or close Ziploc bags or pop tops on cans of ginger ale!"

She spoke ten words I wanted to shove back down her throat as they escaped past her lips: "It's hard to say if the feeling will come back."

I could feel the tears again but pushed them down. I didn't want to hear this, to deal with this, so I pushed everything down to deal with later.

She inspected my toe that was now oozing clear liquid. The right big toenail started to detach from the skin. It had gone from purple to a whitish gray. It looked like the color I imagined a dead body to look like. Deathly Gray. I wondered if I could sell that name to Sherwin Williams for a new paint color.

We reviewed my neutrophil levels. Last week I was at .76 and this week I had only climbed to .89 which was still too low for treatment. I needed to be at 1.0. I was not surprised at how low my levels were. My body was crying out, enough. There was an immediate sense of relief, but I remembered I had one more week scheduled. "Do you think my oncologist will let me stop treatment even though I have only had seven injections of Taxol?"

"He isn't here today so you will be visiting with another oncologist. I can't answer that. He will let you know, but there is a possibility you will be released since you are suffering from neuropathy." I was instantly disappointed to discover my oncologist was not in the office. He advocated for me several weeks ago when I begged for my last treatment with the Red Devil. I knew he wouldn't let me continue with the issues I was having. Who was this new character I was going to meet?

After Rachel departed, another oncologist entered my room. He was a thin man somewhere close to 65, I guessed. His hair was gray and thinning. He wore glasses down on the end of his nose. I imagined he had a full bank account, but his suit appeared to be more like what Al Bundy wore working in a lady's shoe store. His shoulders were littered with dandruff. I decided I wouldn't hold this against him unless he wanted to continue injecting me with poison, then I would go all fashion police on him and let him know he clearly needed an Ermenegildo Zegna suit to be working at this renowned medical center.

"We can't treat you today, so you are going home," he said. "Your neutrophils haven't recovered from your treatment two weeks ago. But first, let's talk about the neuropathy."

He said nerve endings take a while to heal. The best thing for neuropathy is exercising your fingers. I chimed in, "I'm a writer. I write long hand and type a lot!"

"That's perfect," he said. "You can also use a squishy ball or something to work those nerve endings. We don't know and can't guarantee the nerves will heal. They may be damaged for the rest of your life." Those last few words, "for the rest of your life," hung in the air like a thick fog.

"If you were my sister, I would recommend we stop giving you chemo treatments. At this point, the Taxol is doing more harm than good," he said. There was something so beautiful and horrifying about this statement. What else had this poison done to my body?

I was done. Wait. What? I was done! There was no one with me to celebrate. I walked towards the exit with a smile pasted across my face. I walked through the waiting room and called my mother, then Adlai and started sending out a few text messages.

I looked out the large windows in the hallway. There was a light dusting of snow on the ground. Workers below set up Peace Plaza for an annual event called SocialICE. Each year, restaurants created a bar with themed ice sculptures. The bartenders dressed up to match the theme, and they also served specialty drinks. This year, my parents were driving from Missouri to attend. It was Thursday, and they were set to drive on Friday so we could attend the event on Saturday. I was so excited especially since I was finished with chemo. It was going to be a celebration!

That Friday, a massive snowstorm ripped through Iowa which made travel conditions too treacherous for my parents to drive. I was disappointed, but of course I understood. Adlai and I decided to brave the cold weather Saturday evening and continue as planned. We bundled up and drove to Rochester. I was excited for him because this was his first year experiencing this event, whereas I had been a few times in the past with friends.

The temperatures were unbearable as we walked from the car to Peace Plaza. The event had drawn so many people we had to park about six blocks away. Normally, I would have enjoyed the fresh air, but with the temperatures in single digits, and a compromised immune system, the experience was less than desirable.

As Adlai and I neared Peace Plaza, there was a fire pit with a mass of people gathered around it. The first thing Adlai wanted to do was warm up around the fire. I started to whine, "No, I have my nice down coat on. I'll smell like a campfire!" He grabbed my hand and tugged me inside one of the retail stores. I was excited to spend time rifling through the racks full of clothing. He gave me about five minutes to warm up, then we went out to brave the cold and look for a warm drink.

The plaza was so crowded we could barely see any of the bars, let alone get in line for a drink. The crowd was moving at a snail's pace, so he pulled me to the outer edge of the plaza where there were only a few people. In minutes the frigid weather burrowed into my skin, so we ducked inside of one of the hotel lobbies. Both of us agreed this event was not the best place for a cancer patient with a weakened immune system.

By the time we arrived back at the car, my fingers ached. The cold and the neuropathy made my fingers feel like someone hit them with a hammer. The engine turned over and cold air blasted from the dashboard. He turned down the fan until the car heated up. This night was a bust. "Let's find a restaurant. I'm hungry," I said. We found a low-key restaurant away from downtown and celebrated my milestone: My treatments were done. No more chemo!

# Part 4: Radiation

# Consultation

Celebrating the finale of my chemo treatments was short and sweet. My first radiation consultation was scheduled less than two weeks after chemo ended. Before the radiation appointment, I had a follow-up appointment with my plastic surgeon—my six-month post-surgical checkup. The results pleased both of us, and he asked me about chemo, and my remaining treatment plan. We discussed the severity of side effects, mainly neuropathy, and the doctor's choice to stop treatment after seven rounds of Taxol. I mentioned the visit with the radiation oncologist today and wondered if I needed to worry about this phase of the treatment. He brushed off my concerns, and I left his office confident and happy.

Later that morning, I met my friend Sarah in the parking lot of the clinic where I had completed chemo. She baked four types of cookies for me so I could give them to my chemo nurses. I decided to do this mid-way through treatments when I discovered the love and commitment these nurses had for their jobs and their patients, and now it was finally time.

Sarah baked two heaping trays of cookies; my spindly arms could barely hold the weight of them. We walked together to the chemo ward. Upon arrival, I asked for one of my favorite nurses. She came from behind a curtain and flashed a gigantic, toothy smile. She embraced me and said I looked well. I passed one of the trays of cookies to her.

"These are for the nurses. I really appreciate the magnificent care I received from each one of you. "Thank you," I said. Sarah snapped a photo with me, the cookies, and the beautiful nurses that day. My heart fluttered with delight, as a smile spanned from ear to ear. Giving back to the people who helped save my life pumped up my psyche. Happiness washed over my mind, body, and soul like a chrysalis surrounding a soon-to-be butterfly.

Sarah went about her day as I made my way to my next appointment. As I approached the doors to the radiology waiting room, I could see a large group of people huddled around the infamous bell referred to as The Sound of Hope. I heard the bell chime three times and listened to the group of people as they cheered. A bald man stood in the middle of the group dressed in pajama bottoms and a faded green t-shirt. First, I heard laughter and then sniffles as a few guests shed tears.

I stood erect as a tinge of jealousy shot up my spine. I imagined myself standing in front of the bell. I wanted to push the fast forward button on my treatment. I visualized my husband and my parents and family standing around me. One by one the Fitness Friends and other treasured friends gathered around me as I approached the bell. I had to stop my daydreaming to focus and prepare for the recommendations from the radiology oncologist.

The receptionist passed the pager across the desk, and I turned and looked around the waiting room for a chair. Most chairs were taken, and a buzz of conversation filled the air. I picked a chair next to an older couple and while I usually keep one seat between me and the other person in the waiting room, there weren't enough chairs to separate us. I stripped the heavy down coat from around me and set my belongings on the floor, trying to be mindful of their personal space. The artwork along the wall captured my attention immediately. It was a large glass rainbow wall hanging that overwhelmed the white wall. It was waiting for me to make a wish. The rainbow wasn't arched like you see in nature, it was a rainbow of vertical stripes about 15 feet long and five feet tall. The glass rippled along the wall. On one end of the glass, a vivid yellow stripe blended into other warm colors and slowly changed to cool colors and then ended with a bright azure blue. My mind traveled to far-away places. I floated my wish to the glass rainbow. "Please keep me safe, healthy, and strong through this final treatment."

As I waited for my pager to go off, I dug in my purse for my contoured gel hand grip. Adlai found the squeezable gel grip at Scheels and brought it home to soothe my neuropathy. I took it everywhere and tried to will the neuropathy out of my hands. As I squeezed the green gel, my palms became sweaty and my knee bobbed up and down. I felt unprepared and prayed for no major bombs to be dropped on me.

Sweat spread from palms to my armpits and then to my forehead. A woman with a royal blue canvas jacket and a name tag that read Susan approached me and asked if I wanted something to drink. I said, "Yes, I'll have a glass of red wine." She laughed loudly like it was the funniest thing she had ever heard, though I assumed she had heard that line many times before. I settled for apple juice and sucked it down through the mini black straw in about three gulps. Seconds later, my pager vibrated.

D-day, I thought to myself. I repeated in my head, breathe…breathe…breathe. I gave my name and birthdate to the person who called me back, and I stepped on the scale as he jotted down my weight. He led me to a doctor's office and the waiting game started.

I fidgeted with the zipper on my handbag while my eyes darted around the sterile room. I searched for some indication of what was about to happen, but the room was barren. Not even cautionary medical posters on the wall to distract me. The only thing I had to stare at was the patient table with the roll of tissue paper spread from top to bottom.

I took a few deep breaths when a petite Indian woman knocked softly and entered the room. She extended her hand and introduced herself as the senior resident, so I shoved the gel grip into my purse and extended my arm. The gold bracelets on her delicate wrist jingled. My gut turned as a burning sensation flooded my abdomen. I wanted the radiation oncologist listed on my appointment guide. Who was this mysterious woman, and why wasn't the actual doctor here to visit me on my first appointment? A senior resident? Seriously?

She sidestepped pleasantries and explained, "Radiation is a high energy beam used to destroy cancer cells. Because you had cancer in your lymph nodes, we are going to radiate a large area from below the breast mound into your armpit and up to your clavicle." She went on to tell me I would have 25 photon treatments; once a day, five days per week. The doctor chose photon radiation, or the x-ray type of radiation, instead of proton beam radiation because of the location of my cancer. "The proton beam is currently used for breast cancer patients who have cancer located on the left side. We use it to protect the heart from damage, however, there aren't enough studies that show proton beam is safer and more effective, so we will use the most common method, the photon treatment. Besides, the proton beam is considered experimental by many insurance companies."

"Before we start radiation, we will do a simulation to get the most effective treatment set up for you," she continued. This sounded easy, until she slammed me with the side effects of radiation. The photon beam could cause the skin and tissue below the skin to harden. "Since you have already had your surgery, the surgical scar tissue can harden and put pressure on the implant. This is called capsular contraction, and it deforms the shape of the breast and causes significant pain. Many times, an additional surgery is needed to remedy the side effects of radiation."

Hearing the side effects made me furious and second guess radiation treatment. "Wait. I don't understand. I had surgery to remove all the cancer from my breast and lymph nodes. Then I had chemo treatments which is essentially just poison and lymph nodes filter out

Nicole L. Czarnomski

poison. Isn't there plenty of poison in my lymph nodes battling cancer? Why do I need radiation?" I asked.

She told me I was young, and this treatment would increase my life expectancy and would keep me cancer-free.

"Even though the cancer was cut out, there's no way to tell if the cancer spread to more lymph nodes above the breast mound," she said. I went from sad to furious in seconds. It felt like someone slammed me in the gut with a two-by-four. Heat shot through my body, and I could feel my face turn red and the sweat beads cluster underneath my hat.

I yanked the hat off the top of my shiny, bald head and asked, "What if I don't do this?" Before I could let her answer, I exclaimed, "I don't want to be here! I don't want to do this! Why is this happening to me?"

I worked so hard with my physical therapist to get my breasts to look somewhat normal after my reconstructive surgery. I was happy with the results, as happy as I could be with fake boobs. They were perky and plump, and the same size pre-surgery. The scars faded into a purplish-pink hue instead of the startling rouge they were early on.

The pressure inside my tear ducts felt like I had shaken a bottle of sparkling wine and the cork was ready to burst off. Her piercing brown eyes dug holes deep inside of me. She casually set the box of tissues next to me on the desk. My retinas burned. She sat quietly as I plucked tissues from the box and wiped the tears away.

"I understand your frustration," she said softly. "Typically, when radiation is recommended, plastic surgeons start with expanders instead of going straight to implants. Then if there is damage, the expanders are removed and replaced."

Unfortunately, this was not the method my surgeon and general surgeon chose for me. Even though a football-shaped piece of skin was removed during surgery, there was plenty of skin to support C-sized implants. She made me feel like I was stupid and should have known better. Shamed me like a dog who just shredded the contents of the trash.

"I don't want to do this. Just forget about it!" I was about to walk out of the office and face the chances of getting cancer again. I looked at her and said, "This doesn't make sense. I went through nearly five months of chemotherapy. That is poison, and the lymph nodes filter poison from the body. My lymph nodes should be full of chemo, why do they need to be radiated?"

She explained that radiation focused more on the lymphatic system whereas chemo wasn't as direct. (To this day, I don't understand why chemo doesn't fight cancer in the lymph nodes.) She urged me to reconsider and said the nurse would come in to discuss ways to protect the skin from the radiation beams. She dismissed any hesitation I felt for this treatment, confident I would change my mind and acquiesce to the dreaded treatment.

I watched her exit my room with her perfect tweed blazer, angered by her air of superiority and lack of empathy. Nurse Julie entered almost immediately following the fashionista. She was another one of those people who whispered, but this time I knew why she whispered to me. She sensed my longing to scream. I didn't want to scream at her, but I wanted to scream at the situation.

Nurse Julie discussed scheduling the simulation appointment and gave me the information about this process. She dismissed my utter disgust for this treatment, and told me my team was the A-team, and they were amazing! She talked to me like I had decided to go forward with this stupid treatment.

Nicole L. Czarnomski

"Wait, I don't want to do this!" I exclaimed. Her brows raised and eyes widened.

"Why? This is an important piece of your treatment." I explained my concerns about the implants. I also expressed my displeasure with the senior resident. In a whisper, she repeated my last two sentences to make sure she heard me correctly.

"Yeah, you heard me. Now, can I leave?"

"Let me see if I can find the senior consultant before we make any decisions," she said.

The radiology oncologist entered my room soon after Julie left. She was tall and slender and spoke in a slow, soft and direct manner as if she were hand picking each word before it rolled off her tongue. The senior resident followed her into my room, and I could barely contain the need to holler expletives at her.

The senior consultant went through the importance of radiation one more time and said I shouldn't be concerned about my implants. She assured me that the treatment plan would do little damage to the implant. "The skin and scar tissue around the implants could see the most damage," she said matter of fact. "Each person reacts differently to treatment." There were no guarantees, but she seemed hopeful. "Mepitel is a new product we've been using to help with radiation side effects. It's a thin barrier to protect skin from the harsh radiation treatments. The nurse will apply a thin layer of plastic over the radiated area. It doesn't protect what's underneath the skin, only the surface of the skin."

After bouncing around between anger, sadness, anger again, frustration, confusion, and more anger, I finally acquiesced. I scheduled a simulation appointment, begrudgingly moving forward with the last major phase of my treatment.

Before my radiation simulation appointment, I met with my oncologist regarding endocrine therapy and follow up from my last chemo treatment. He asked about the neuropathy in my hands and feet. I told him the neuropathy was still evident, but I felt like it may be getting a little better. I told him I was still using the squishy, gel grip as often as possible.

We then discussed the last phase of my treatment, Tamoxifen. He explained how it would suppress the function of the ovaries, and if my body reacted well, he wanted to consider additional medication to further suppress the function of my ovaries.

"I would like to finish radiation treatments before we start the Tamoxifen. Please allow me to do one step at a time," I said with a hint of desperation. He agreed and said he would go ahead and submit my prescription to the pharmacy.

"Start taking this pill immediately following radiation, and I will schedule another appointment with you about one month after you start taking it. I want to know how your body reacts to this," he said, his tone more serious than usual.

After our discussion, he said he needed blood work done prior to starting Tamoxifen. "I want to see if your body will metabolize the drug before you start taking it," he said. "I will advise you if your body rejects the drug. Otherwise, begin taking it after radiation as planned." I agreed and made the appointment.

Nicole L. Czarnomski

Radiation simulation was scheduled one week after my first appointment with the senior resident. My friend Denise, the yoga instructor, waited for me as we had planned the night before at her yoga class. Though most of her classes left me feeling relaxed and healthy, last night's class was the polar opposite; I felt lousy. After many downward facing dogs, my strength waned, and I struggled to make sense of radiation. I couldn't rid my mind of this devastating new treatment. While I rolled my mat and grabbed my block to put on the shelf, my friend Kelly said, "Your sparkle seems a little lackluster this evening. Are you okay?" Without hesitation, I broke into an uncontrollable, sloppy, heaving mess. Yogis gathered around me as tears and snot poured from my face. Between each heaving breath, I explained my fear, anger, and sadness regarding the next leg of my journey. The choice my plastic surgeon made to go straight to implants instead of expanders left me questioning his thought process. I tried to express my fear to the six ladies now gathered around me, hugging me. My crying fit paused briefly, and Denise asked if I wanted moral support at my simulation appointment. I agreed to her kind offer and told her to meet me at the clinic the next afternoon.

Denise and I huddled on a bench together, and when I heard my name called, she asked if I wanted her to come with me. I agreed with an emphatic Yes! We sat in the office together as nurse Julie reviewed the simulation with me. Denise held my hand the whole time ignoring my sweaty palms, her grip tender, yet supportive. Once the discussion was over, Denise let go of my hand, gave me a big hug and went back to her office. There was nothing more she could do for me; I had to do the simulation alone.

The nurse led me to a room so I could change out of my blouse and into a long cotton gown. When I walked into the simulation room, there were three women waiting for me. Each one tried to make small talk while they prepped me for the simulation. Conversing with these three ladies reminded me of an awkward first date.

One of the women asked me to disrobe. Another woman held a small, blue rectangular piece of cloth the size of a placemat in front of my breasts, a cheap gesture of modesty. I wondered if the radiation therapists were thinking about the size I chose. I wanted to interject something about the size C cup being an original size, but I didn't know what to say. I felt awkward and jealous standing in front of three women who most likely still had their natural breasts. It was the first time I realized just how fake my boobs were. The room was freezing, and I found myself yearning to have pointy, hard nipples, but there was nothing but light purplish pink scars where my nipples once resided.

The three therapists helped position me on a large MRI looking machine. They made sure to keep my breasts cloaked with the small blue cloth. After I was lying down, one of the therapists covered my legs with a warm blanket to stop my teeth from chattering.

Both of my arms were extended each clutching an overhead bar as I lay on my back. The senior consultant graced me with her presence today, and her senior resident followed closely behind her like a duckling. All of the staff spoke using medical terms, so I tuned out. My eyes wandered around the cold and sterile room. White walls and fluorescent lights created an eerie horror movie-like environment. Five women hovered over my body like sharks circling their prey.

"Lower your left arm and position it by your side," the senior consultant said in her slow, soft voice. I moved my arm. In an even softer voice I heard her say, "Yes, I believe it will work with the left arm down. I want to minimize the amount of radiation going to the left breast mound, heart, and lungs." My thoughts accelerated like a race car on the straightaway. Damage to the other side as well? I imagined a whole new surgery for both lefty and righty. When would this surgery take place? In a few weeks…months…years? I redirected my thoughts. One day at a time, Nicole, one day at a time.

Nicole L. Czarnomski

Part two of the simulation left me with tattoos. There were three dots the size of freckles tattooed onto my stomach to help with placement of a small box. Once the tattoos were in place, they secured a small box to my abdomen and put clear circular stickers on my diaphragm to help with placement.

The box on my abdomen helped measure my breath. I had to hold my breath for 15-20 seconds to keep from moving. If I didn't inhale and hold the oxygen in my lungs, or if I wiggled, it could damage other parts of the body that didn't need to be radiated, specifically my lungs. I felt a stinging in my eyes. Manic thoughts pulsated through my brain. Damaged left and right breast. Damaged lungs. Hardened skin tissue. Hardened scar tissue. Damage. Damage. Damage. Just before the tear ran down the side of my face, I told myself, That's enough. These people are here to save your life. Let them do their job.

One of the therapists gave me a pair of glasses that looked like virtual reality goggles. The viewing screen inside the glasses had a white background with a thick immobile blue line toward the top and a yellowish moving bar at the bottom. When I took a breath, the yellowish bar shot up and hovered over the blue band creating a greenish band. My job was to hold the green bar in place until a technician over the loudspeaker said breathe. Finally, something my art major brain could understand.

The final piece of this simulation was to create a radiation bolus. The radiation therapist heated a large sheet of Barbie pink plastic until it became malleable. She positioned the pink plastic over my right breast. The material was hot, but not to the point of burning the skin. The pink plastic melted around my breast mound as the therapist molded and shaped it like she was potter sculpting clay. After the plastic cooled, she removed it and trimmed off the excess. There before my eyes, an impression of my right breast, a work of art. My plastic

169

surgeon would be proud. The bolus would be used during each treatment to target the specific area to be radiated.

Nicole L. Czarnomski

# Beamin' My Boobies

The following Monday, I arrived back at the clinic for my first radiation treatment. Prior to treatment, I undressed from the waist up and cloaked my body in a gown. I opened the gown and nurse Julie applied the Mepitel film to the right breast and armpit. It had the consistency of saran wrap. This magic paper was going to save my skin from the harsh radiation beams. I was skeptical that something so flimsy could protect my skin, but I trusted the medical professionals.

The nurse guided me towards the radiation room and asked me to wait for the radiation therapist. I stood in a hall half-dressed peering down at the grayish tile floor diverting my gaze from the random people walking by. My gown was void of strings but had a few snaps in the front. With the gawkers passing by, I wished I would have fastened the snaps on my gown.

A radiation therapist stepped out of a room about five feet away from me. Her presence jolted my body as I gasped for air. She asked if I was Mrs. Czarnomski. I said yes, and she introduced herself as Jenna. Cheryl followed closely behind Jenna, and she too introduced herself. When I walked into the room, I saw the same MRI looking machine from last week and wished this appointment was a simulation rather than the real thing.

Next to the large machine, Alex greeted me with a professional hello. Shit. A guy? I thought to myself. I had to expose my imposters to another guy. Embarrassment clung to me like a sloth in a tree. I wondered if he thought I was stupid too. Stupid for going straight to implants instead of expanders.

I thought about asking for all females next time, but soon realized he was professional and good at his job. He was the one therapist who always remembered to put my Barbie pink bolus under the warm blanket on my knee, so it had time to warm up before he placed it on my breast.

While Cheryl and Jenna helped me disrobe, Alex retrieved the warm blanket and covered me from the waist down and made sure my bolus was heating up. Tom Petty's song, American Girl, played on the stereo system in my room. Alex asked if classic rock was okay, and I said yes hoping I wouldn't hit panic like I did months ago during my first breast MRI.

The therapists helped me on to the big machine and guided my right arm towards the handlebar over my head. I extended my hand and found the familiar bar to clutch for my specific treatment plan. I gripped the bar like I was about to ride the Tilt-a-Whirl at the county fair. I laid on a lightweight sheet, so my body wasn't touching the actual machine. Jenna instructed me to relax. "I need to reposition you, and I am going to do so by pulling on the sheet below you," she said. I doubted her ability to move this 147-pound girl by pulling on a sheet.

I inhaled and exhaled. She scooted me a few centimeters. Alex confirmed the new positioning, and he taped the magic box to my abdomen. He gave me a pair of goggles, the ones where I blend yellow and blue to make green. When they were fastened to my head, I could see the colored bars again, and I knew what to do.

Before they left the room, Jenna said, "We are going to take x-rays first to ensure we radiate the appropriate areas. Then, we will complete the radiation treatment." Alex secured the bolus to my right breast and the three of them walked out of my room as I hummed along with Tom Petty.

Within seconds I heard Jenna say over a speaker, "Take a deep breath." I inhaled like it was my last breath. I hoped the radiation beams wouldn't hit my lungs. I held my breath for only a few seconds when I heard Jenna say breathe. The single panel above my chest moved to the left. Shoot! That was the x-ray, I remembered. I wasted one good deep breath for a simple x-ray. I doubted my ability to take another deep breath as good as the first one.

I heard the words, take a deep breath, so I complied, sending the yellow bar up to the blue, making the perfect green. A loud buzzing sound filled the room and startled me. The sound made me picture a mass frenzy running down the halls of the clinic followed by intruder alert…intruder alert sounding over the speakers. "You can breathe," said Jenna.

The loud buzzing sound stopped, and I let the air out of my lungs. I felt my chest lower. The screen rotated around my body. Another x-ray was taken, followed by instructions to breathe, then the loud buzzing sound and exhale. The screen continued to rotate multiple times. After the last breath, a smiley face and the word Good Job! popped up on the screen inside the glasses, making me giggle. Round one was done in a matter of 20 minutes. I hadn't even realized they started the radiation treatment. Radiation seemed harmless.

The three therapists came back into my room and helped me off the machine. Cheryl grabbed my gown off the coat hanger. She held it as I slid my arms through the arm holes. Jenna led me back to my changing room and explained the process for the next five weeks. "When you arrive, you will receive the pager. When it goes off, walk back to this dressing room, put on a robe and one of us will come find you for treatment," she said. The A-team had impressed me today.

For the next five weeks, I continued to work 32 hours a week. The schedule exhausted me, but I couldn't fall below 32 hours, or I would lose my health insurance, or worse, a job I loved. I battled through my daily tasks like a wounded soldier. My mind functioned below my normal acuity. I found myself in mid-sentence searching for the appropriate word which seemed to be flying around me like a pesky fly—always out of reach. It embarrassed me.

During radiation treatments, my only solace was getting to leave the office at 3:00–3:30 p.m. each day to walk to my appointment. The walk took about 35 minutes, and it was rejuvenating, it kept me sane. In the evening, if I had the energy, I quieted my mind with 20-30 minutes of yoga on YouTube.

The countdown to completion started on Friday after my first full week of radiation treatments. The receptionist snapped a picture of me in front of the infamous bell. I held a sign stating 5 DOWN!! By Friday, I was rocking these treatments. I befriended the radiation therapists because of their awesomeness, professionalism, and they laughed at my cheesy jokes! Their ability to care for me and my needs was evident from day one. They too were giving me another day to live, so no matter how frightening the side effects of radiation sounded, I wanted to make the best of my situation. I showed up to my treatments every day with a smile. I laughed with the A-team like I laughed about farts with my husband.

Each week, I met with my radiation oncologist and one of the nurses. The Mepitel across my right breast was replaced each week because it wore off in a few places, though I was surprised at how well it held up. It adhered to my skin even with daily showers. My doctor believed my skin looked healthy and things were progressing nicely. The nurse who replaced my Mepitel that week said it was not uncommon for plastic surgeons to go straight to implants even though a patient needs radiation. The effects of radiation can also make the expander transfer surgery difficult. It was comforting to hear…sort of.

By week two, righty was beginning to feel full and tight and I wondered if I had capsular contracture already. The mound felt like someone duct taped a grapefruit to my chest well. My new physical therapist, Jenny, assured me that the swelling was because of the lymphatic fluid and irritation of the radiation beams. My breast was not ruined after two weeks of treatment, just sore.

Radiation felt a lot like the movie "Groundhog's Day"—repetitive. I woke up, went to work, walked to radiation, went through treatment, went home, ate dinner, and fell asleep each evening at 7:30. During week three, I changed my route from work to the clinic. I took side streets and noticed well-groomed older homes. I daydreamed about buying an old house and renovating it with my handy husband. I wondered how different my life would have been if I would have continued with the interior design program, my first major, in undergraduate instead of changing my mind five times.

I rehashed my past as if it were a movie reel. I wondered why I couldn't commit to anything in my twenties, from relationships to college majors to jobs. My career trajectory had changed multiple times. I dated a handful of guys before finally meeting the man who became my husband at age 34. Happy that I waited for the right man to marry, I was left wondering if my dissatisfaction with life for so many years gave me cancer.

As I walked, thoughts about living and dying permeated through me. Thoughts of dying brought me to tears many times during my walks to treatment, so I redirected them often. Some days, I chanted softly. "I am strong. I am healthy. I am cancer-free. I am strong. I am healthy. I am cancer-free." Before long, I could feel my lips change from a quiver to a smile. I learned that your attitude is always about your perspective.

By the time I reached the clinic for radiation, depression and fear were fleeting thoughts, and I smiled and laughed with the A-team. The whole radiation team became part of my cancer family. The therapists started asking me if I walked and if the weather was nice. They wanted to know if I was cooking dinner, and what I was making.

Like the chemo nurses, I felt the same way about the radiation therapists. I wanted them all in my circle of friends.

Week four was a turning point. Thoughts of death were replaced with gratitude. I lived life with gusto. During week four, I smiled for the camera every day with a sign counting down to how many treatments remained. The reception team looked forward to my goofy smiles and giddy attitude when they snapped the picture. I couldn't help it; I was so damn excited! 10 MORE! 9 MORE! 8 MORE! Cancer was going down!

Nearing the end of treatment, I decided I wanted to give a speech at the bell ringing. I used my walk to try and remember who I wanted to thank. This was overwhelming on two levels. First, there were so many people to thank the speech may become lengthy. Second, I started to cry at the thought of all the love I received on this journey. I rehearsed my speech each day and took notes when I got home so I wouldn't forget anyone.

With two treatments left, my Fitness Friend Kellie baked pink cake pops for my radiation team. She dropped them off early that morning before I left for work. The pops were adorable—pink and perfect for my breast cancer journey. After my treatment that day, a nurse, who held the cake pops, and therapist gathered around me while I held my sign by the bell. Only one more treatment to go.

By the time my last treatment arrived, my stomach fluttered like a flag blowing in the wind. My parents drove from Missouri, my cousin and his wife drove in from the Minneapolis area and many friends from the surrounding area came to watch me ring that bell.

Nicole L. Czarnomski

My last treatment was Friday, April 6, 2018. I took the day off from work, and my mom accompanied me to a couple of appointments I had while my husband and father were out running errands.

We gathered at the clinic around 4 p.m. that afternoon. Mom and I met up with some of my Fitness Friends and Sarah had a princess crown for me to wear. The crown set atop my head that had new sprouts of hair coming in. So far, all I could tell is my hair color was going to be dark. It was not yet long enough to determine if my new hair would be curly or straight. I had many people tell me that hair often comes in curly after chemotherapy.

When I went back for my last treatment, the waiting room was quiet. My pager went off, and the flag in my gut continued to flutter. I met with my doctor. She told me the surface of my skin would begin to feel the effects of radiation next week. I could expect a rash, or the skin tissue may be raw. "If there are open wounds, contact us immediately so we can prescribe an antibiotic. The open wound can create an infection in the implant," my doctor said. After she schooled me on things to look for, I asked her the question. "Can I say I am cancer-free?"

She looked at me and said, "As of today, there are no traces of cancer in your system." A slight chill rippled my spine, and then the biggest smile I have had since all of this started crossed my face.

"Thank you," I said.

I went back to the room for my last radiation treatment. When treatment was finished, I shook with such fervor my teeth chattered. The therapists all wished me well. I was presented with a small pin to show the finale of my treatment.

After I dressed and tossed my robe into the canvas bag one last time, I checked my face in the mirror, and smiled again noticing the small dimple on my right freckled cheek. I walked down the hall to the waiting room, listening to the clunk of my boot heels on the tile. When I arrived in the waiting room, dozens of people stood waiting for me, people I didn't expect to see. I ran around the room hugging people, thanking them for coming, and giggling with delight. I pulled myself together and found my list of people to thank. Sarah used my phone so I could post a Facebook live video. I stepped to the front of the room, next to the bell, and the room fell silent. Sarah pointed at me when the video went live, and I started my speech.

It went something like this:

Nine months and three days ago, I was diagnosed with stage 3 breast cancer that had spread to my lymph nodes. I went through a double mastectomy with reconstructive surgery, nearly five months of chemotherapy, until the side effects were too much for my body, and 25 radiation treatments. And today, my radiology oncologist said it's safe to say I am cancer-free!

As the tears formed in my eyes, I started with my husband. I thanked him for wiping away the many tears I had shed along this journey and for making me laugh even when I didn't think I had a smile inside. I thanked my parents for their many trips from Missouri, along with their love and support from afar. The constant boobie boxes I received in the mail were appreciated. I thanked the rest of my family, and then on to my Fitness Friends. I thanked new and old friends from near and far. I thanked local businesses for the successful fundraiser. My final statement in my speech was this:

Although I may have been physically alone many times in this journey, I have never, ever once been truly alone on this journey. Thank you all. I love you with my whole heart.

I looked at Sarah cueing her to stop the video, but I had forgotten to ring the bell. Everyone was whispering, "Ring the bell. Ring the bell."

"Oh yes!" I exclaimed. "The bell. Since I went through nine months of this, I am ringing the bell nine times." And I did. I rang that bell loud and proud nine times, turned to the audience and threw my hands in the air.

Adlai embraced me. Today, happy tears were flowing. I hugged so many people and thanked them for their support. Afterward, we met at Twigs, one of my favorite restaurants in Rochester, for a celebration.

I was finished with treatment. Now what?

# Part 5: The Aftermath

Nicole L. Czarnomski

# Feel the Burn

Less than one week after radiation, the skin on my right breast expressed her anger. A bright red band surfaced around the edges of the breast mound. It was the worst sunburn ever. A red rash with white papules formed under the breast mound and spread around the breast, up my sternum, and then back around the top of the mound. The rash blazed hot and angry, uncomfortable and itchy. Each day, I selected a loose-fitting tank top instead of a bra because of the discomfort I felt along my chest.

When I called the doctor, she wasn't surprised. She recommended Vanicream and Aquaphor for the irritated skin tissue. She also sent in a prescription for Mometasone Furoate. She believed the rash was radiation dermatitis. Within a week the rash calmed down, so I stopped using the creams. Days later, it returned, and so did the reapplication of Mometasone and Aquaphor.

Using Aquaphor was problematic. It had the consistency of Vaseline. I purchased gauze pads to cover the sticky, goopy breast mound, and I tried to protect my clothes from the gelatinous goop, but it wasn't easy. Without a bra, there wasn't anything securing the gauze to my skin, and I didn't want tape anywhere around the site. I had visions of the gauze slipping out from under my shirt like the poor ladies that leave the bathroom with toilet paper streaming from the bottom of their shoes. Maybe duct tape would have been a good option.

The rash began to go away for the second time, and I noticed renewed energy levels. It was almost May, so the weather was perfect for outdoor running. I laced up my running shoes, squished my girls into a compression bra and hit the pavement for one of my first runs post-treatment.

I knew the importance of building up the time and mileage rather than running for 30 straight minutes. I started with a five-minute walk and a 30 second run. And again, five minutes of walking, then 30 seconds of running. Over the next few weeks, I increased the run time and decreased the walk time. I had some concerns about my breasts at first. Would running be painful? Would the chest muscle really keep the implant in place? The more I ran, I realized there was nothing to worry about, and my fear subsided. It wasn't painful at all, and I was happy I chose to have my implants inserted under the chest wall. The only downside was that I could contract the chest muscles and my boobs moved up and down like a body builder. Not real sexy, but I felt confident the implants were going to stay put.

Sadly, within the first week of running, a rash fierier than the first blazed across my right breast again halting my exercise routine. I applied Vanicream and Mometasone and hoped for relief. I called my radiation oncologist and let her know that my rash had returned for the third time. She scheduled an appointment to examine the skin's reaction. In the meantime, no running.

My rash stumped my doctor. She stared at my boob looking for an answer to burst from the incision. Perplexed was her term. She contacted the dermatology team and scheduled an appointment for the next day.

The dermatologist's English accent decorated the room like party favors. She had a thin frame, and blonde hair and an enviable creamy complexion. I desperately wanted her healthy, milky skin on my boobs instead of the lipstick-colored red rash. She recommended a biopsy, but I put the brakes on that idea. I requested more observation and a stronger medication. The thought of another procedure on my right breast felt like an assault. The old girl suffered enough, the last thing I wanted was a puncture wound followed by a gnarly bruise unfurling on Righty.

She asked if one of her colleagues could examine my breast when I declined the biopsy. "Sure," I said, "Show anybody you want. Just make the rash go away."

She returned with a tall skinny man who looked barely old enough to be in college much less a physician at the clinic. He was wearing a bright blue polyester vest, and I wondered if he worked in IT. Awkward. I didn't mean just anybody. Why is the IT guy here to look at my boobs? The dermatologist introduced him as a doctor; I guessed he didn't have to wear the proverbial white coat over his street clothes. I flashed my boob with trepidation still not able to process his status as a doctor.

"This looks like radiation related erythema," he said matter of fact. "Continue with the Mometasone and come back in one month, and we can re-evaluate the skin tissue."

The dermatologist invited the professional clinic photographer into my room to take a picture of the rouge-colored rash on my chest. Righty was famous now with the Mayo paparazzi photographing her. I wondered if she would get a building or statue named after her. I left the office disappointed they couldn't do more but comforted that it wasn't anything worse.

A week later, the rash dissipated. I continued with the steroid cream until the tube was empty. I waited another week and started my exercise routine. I alternated running with exercise DVDs. I perspired to the modification track on the Insanity DVDs, and I included weight intensive videos. Each video made my heart thump so hard I thought it would shatter my rib cage.

During college, and the few years after graduation was the only time I remember being more out of shape. My inner athlete was lost inside self-deprecating thoughts. When I looked in the mirror, all I could see was fat even though my shoulder blades protruded farther than my breasts. I often wondered if all those negative thoughts about my body caught up to me in the form of cancer.

As I continued with my new exercise routine post-breast cancer treatments, I selected a video for strength training. To be a stronger runner, I needed to re-tone my soft muscles. During one of the exercises, I lunged backward off my aerobics step and when I pulled my leg forward to drive my knee up, a shot of pain crippled my lower back. I froze, grabbing at my back as if my hands could halt the pain.

I iced it, heated it, rested it and babied it, but my back continued to hurt. I even tried regular chiropractic care for the first time, but this pain continued for weeks. Exercise was now on the back burner. I was struggling to understand the abilities of my post-cancer body. My lymphedema physical therapist prescribed a few stretches and ordered an x-ray after four-weeks of constant back pain. This x-ray revealed the beginning of arthritis in my hips but nothing unusual to cause the intense back pain.

I discovered several videos on YouTube for lower back pain and sciatica. I stretched two to three times every day. This injury took more than six weeks to heal. By week seven, I laced up my running shoes for a third time since my treatment ended. And this time, I was on the road to recovery. Now, I could be the girl I was before cancer. Or so I thought.

At work, I became the lone ranger in the marketing department. My supervisor landed a wonderful new position at another company, and while happy for her, it cramped my recovery schedule. Thankfully, our new executive director was incredibly supportive while I tried to keep up with the daily tasks associated with both mine and her roles.

During this time, I received a large bill from the clinic. When I called the clinic, they said the insurance company didn't pay for a test my oncologist ordered. I was baffled because I had met my deductible in January with my chemotherapy treatments. To make matters worse, the insurance company never informed me of the denied claim. Upon further investigation, I learned they considered the test experimental. My oncologist ordered this blood test to ensure my body could metabolize Tamoxifen. I had already started taking this prescription, and the insurance company paid for the drug, but not the test to ensure it was okay for my body. I was dumbfounded.

For three straight months, I went back and forth between the clinic and the insurance company trying to get the denial appealed. The insurance company sent me a complaint form but neglected to tell me the form started the appeal process. I thought it was literally a complaint form to express my displeasure with the insurance company. It was literally five months into the dispute, I realized the complaint form started the appeal process, and I needed to fill out the document and send it to the insurance company to get the appeal process moving.

My patience dwindled like a mother fighting with her teenage daughter. I had held down my job during this illness, managed a healthy marriage, stayed somewhat healthy despite the cancer, started an exercise regimen, but now, this fight with the insurance company had me groveling on the floor.

Life continued even though the appeal process moved at a glacial pace. My six-month post chemo appointment was scheduled in late August of 2018; my body shuddered as the elevator chimed and the doors opened to the familiar floor. Anxiety took over. Thoughts of needles, poison, and cancer throbbed in my head. Was it possible to have PTSD over the tenth floor of a building? I patrolled the waiting room looking for clues as to how my first post-chemo appointment would go. I found nothing but the same black and white photos that adorned the walls during my treatment.

When my name was called, it was like a firing pin smacking the rim of a bullet. My body shook. The nice woman who called my name, measured my height and weight. I was disgusted when she announced 5'7" and 162 pounds—a mere four pounds lighter than my heaviest weight ever back in 2006 when I started my master's program.

Since my treatments ended in April, I had gained 15 pounds. Eight of those pounds I had lost over the course of chemo, but the other seven were extra weight from eating whatever I wanted.

Wading through the depressing news about my weight, I followed the young woman down the hall to my private room to await my breast exam. When my oncologist entered the room, I welcomed his warm smile and wished every doctor had his positive mannerisms. "Look at your hair, Nicole!" He may have been as excited as I was to see my hair growing back. It was soft like bunny fur. Part of my daily routine was touching the top of my head just to feel its softness and to celebrate its return. My hair was kind of an ashy color when it returned which was typical. I guess I was more surprised that there were no curls or color changes.

He then asked about the neuropathy in my hands and feet. I grinned and flashed the dimple on my cheek at him. "It's gone!" I said. It had stopped mid-way through my radiation treatments. "I am able to open jars, Ziploc bags, and pop tops again."

We went on to discuss the test for Tamoxifen being deemed as experimental. He was appalled and said he would write a letter to go along with my appeal paperwork. We also discussed my side effects from the pill. I blamed my weight gain on the Tamoxifen, to which he said, "You look great, Nicole. You appear to be very healthy." I thanked him and remembered my grandmother saying I was built like a brick shithouse a couple of months ago. Apparently, that was a compliment back in the days of Marilyn Monroe, but it didn't feel like one to me.

"Oh, I'm having hot flashes too," I said it like it was an afterthought. My good-natured oncologist was not in the least bit worried about hot flashes or the excess weight I had gained.

After our conversation, my oncologist asked me to disrobe to check my breasts. "You can step behind the curtain, and put on the gown," he said.

"It's okay. I'm not modest anymore," I said as I whipped off my top and climbed on the examination table, thankful my injured back was on the mend. He completed a breast exam. I felt awkward when he touched my right breast, she was like a softball stuck to my chest after radiation treatments damaged her. The cording in my underarm was taut like a body builder's flexed muscles. "No new lumps. This is good, Nicole."

I could feel my shoulders fall away from my ears. I hadn't realized the tension I held throughout my body since leaving the waiting room. In a matter of 30 minutes, I passed my breast exam, and my oncologist was going to write an appeal for me in hopes of getting the insurance company to pay for the test. I was relieved. Now, what to do about the extra weight?

# My Raison D'être

My exercise program progressed through September—running, yoga, and light weight training. Each week I grew stronger, so I pushed my physical limitations. By mid-September I jogged in two to three-minute increments several days a week and even managed to maintain this regimen while we vacationed with friends in Cape Cod. A vacation was not going to shove me off course.

While I waited for the insurance company, I marveled at my success. This brick shithouse had lost five freeloading pounds from that summer. By October, I progressed from running 10 minutes straight, to 15, and then 30. Running for 30 straight minutes put me in a position to participate in an organized 5k before the end of the year. Running a 5K the same year I finished treatment seemed like the perfect goal for this one-time athlete.

As I prepared for the 5K, the insurance company finally received all the correct paperwork to start the appeal and within days, a flood of paperwork arrived in the mail. I succeeded! The appeal process was underway. They had 45 days to hold a hearing to decide if the test was experimental.

Since I wanted to run an organized race, I thought it would be fun to have a friend go along. I invited my Fitness Friend Liz to join me, and we were poised to register for a run scheduled at the end of November. This run, my raison d'être, was going to be the grand finale of this book. I wanted to show myself and other cancer patients and survivors that I was leaving cancer in the dust, but my fragile lower back had other plans.

In early November, I completed a rigorous abdominal routine, and a couple of days later my lower back ached. I surrendered to the pain and took a couple of days off from exercising. Less than five days later, it felt like a hammer struck my spine. The nerve pain in my glute and ankle felt like it was sizzling over a BBQ pit. I tried stretching, going to a chiropractor, water walking in a 90-degree warm-water pool, and mentally sending love and support to my lower back. My workouts atrophied along with my injured back. The realization that my body wasn't going to recover as quickly as I wanted post-cancer was difficult to swallow. I contemplated pushing through and running the 5k anyway, but at what cost? Could I do more harm than good? My answer was yes, and I broke the news to my friend. I reminded myself that I had run the 5k over and over during the month of October and even though it wasn't an organized event with a medal and t-shirt waiting for me at the finish line, it called for a celebration!

My husband and I took a short road trip to Milwaukee, Wisconsin, a mini celebration of my success and our love. We celebrated my renewed strength and energy and the bond we had developed over the last year trying not to focus on the pain I was feeling. My body was still healing, waiting for the cocoon to open so I could blossom into the person I was supposed to become post-cancer. I was in between, not yet the beautiful butterfly. I tried to be gentle and kind and love her unconditionally because she was the only body I had. Some days it was hard to look at myself and wonder if my curves were too curvy, but the post-cancer woman whose flower petals were beginning to open reminded the inner critic to shut-up and be grateful for those bodacious curves. I owned those curves!

We enjoyed the trip to Milwaukee, but it wreaked havoc on my back. Pain traveled through my right glute, hip, and my right ankle during the four-hour car ride. The more pain I felt, the more I stretched, and the more aggravated my nerves became. When I returned to work the following Monday, my new supervisor recommended another chiropractor. His methods were gentler than the first two chiropractors I tried, but in the end, my back was still in pain.

The severity of my lower back pain kept us from driving to Missouri for Thanksgiving. When chatting with my friend Katie and her sister Kellie, both Fitness Friends, they asked Adlai and me to join their family for the holiday. "It's a little crazy because there are so many people, but that's how we like it," said Katie. Grateful for the invitation, we made the 15-minute trek to her parent's house. When we arrived, the house was packed with people and food. Everyone welcomed us and made sure we were comfortable. Mama Mic gave us a tour of her home and allowed us to weave our way into her family. We ate and talked and laughed until we departed late afternoon.

I had grown to love the new hair appearing all over my body—even the peach fuzz on my face. The hair on top of my head had been cut a few times since it started growing in and it came in dark brown. I was in love with my new 'do! For the first time ever in my history of haircuts I loved my hair. I loved how quickly it took me to wash it, dry it, and style it. It was straight and a lovely dark walnut color. This new style and color felt true to who I was, so I embraced it and kept the brown pixy cut.

My eyebrows returned, but they were thin and still needed to be drawn with a brow pencil. At first, I experimented with a couple of different ways to draw in thicker brows. I tried thin pencils first and found it didn't give my brows enough visibility. At the recommendation of my stylist Corey, she told me to try brown eye shadow and a tiny angled brush. I had a hard time making them perfect with either one of these methods. Corey reminded me that the brows are sisters and not twins. She said, "It's okay if they don't look exactly alike." I finally settled on a chubby pencil slightly lighter than my walnut hair color.

Nicole L. Czarnomski

Losing eyelashes was the most difficult part of hair loss for me. Not having eyelashes made me look sick and not just I have the flu, but truly sick. To make matters worse, eyelashes were the last to return. I had hoped to find something to help them along. My Fitness Friend Carrie, also a Rodan and Fields rep, told me about Lash Boost, so immediately following treatments, I started using it. The Lash Boost was incredible! My lashes came back thicker and longer than I had ever seen. It felt amazing to have hair again, and I was grateful I didn't have to go through another winter without hair.

# Oh, My Aching Back

The week following Thanksgiving proved to be brutal; I practically crawled into my lymphedema physical therapy session. My back and leg pain were so severe it felt like someone was chipping at my glute and ankle with ice picks. My physical therapist wanted to take me to the emergency room, but I declined and said it would go away as soon as the Ibuprofen kicked in. I toughed it out.

After spending the entire month of November using extra-strength Tylenol and Ibuprofen round-the-clock, I succumbed to the pain. In early December, Adlai and I were on our way to the grocery store. I sat in the front seat with a grimace etched across my face, moaning like a mighty tiger in mid-roar.

"That's enough! I am taking you to the emergency room. This cannot go on." As he pulled into the hospital drive, I could barely get out of the truck. The transporter met me with a wheelchair and rolled me into the hospital as Adlai parked the vehicle.

Pain seared down my leg while the receptionist checked me in. Thankfully they had an open room, and a nurse plunged an IV into the vein of my left arm. As I described the pain and the original injury, Dilaudid, an opioid, gushed through my body. Bile boiled in my stomach.

"Oh God, get me an anti-nausea medication and the trash can! I'm about to vomit! Hurry up!" I scolded the nurse. As quickly as it came, the nausea subsided with the medication, and I soon felt like my body was floating up in the clouds, not a care in the world.

A doctor arrived in my room while I laid in bed trying to relax. He asked about my situation, and I described the first injury in August, and the x-ray showing nothing more than arthritis. I explained the six-week healing process and went on to tell him about my rigorous exercise regimen I started back in September. Then the long car ride to Milwaukee shoved my pain onto a ledge only to be kicked off into burning pit of lava. The excruciating pain was chronic and nothing could soothe it.

My doctor asked about incontinence. He tested the strength of my legs, pushing, pulling asking me to resist the pressure each time. He pricked both legs and feet with a needle to ensure I had feeling in my lower extremities. "Any tingling or numbness?"

"No," I said wearily. I answered correctly to all his questions and passed all the tests. This meant no emergency surgery. The doctor ordered a CT scan of my back. This scan showed an L4-L5 disc protrusion causing moderate to advanced spinal canal narrowing. I spent eight hours in the E.R., and because the pain never subsided, they admitted me to the hospital.

Because I was a cancer patient, I was sent to another location of the hospital. I rode in an ambulance and all I could think about was my insurance. The insurance company denied the appeal even after my oncologist wrote a letter and attached medical documentation to back up his request for the Tamoxifen test. I felt my concern for riding in the ambulance was warranted. When I asked the paramedic if it would be covered by insurance, he kindly told me everything would be fine. The hospital owned the ambulance, so I would not be billed. And he was right.

That evening, a nurse wheeled me into a private room, to which I asked, "Am I going to be billed for a private room?" The nurse seemed puzzled at the question. "We only have private rooms here. Insurance will cover your stay," she said. "I'll have the social worker come and speak to you in the morning if that will put your mind at ease."

Sleep evaded me the first night. Although the Dilaudid wrestled with my REM cycles and had me begging for sleep, the nurse's nightly checks every two hours to monitor my vitals kept me awake. I welcomed the visits when they brought more pain pills. It was the best I had felt in weeks. The following morning, a team of doctors greeted me at 8:30. Two pain specialists, two physical therapists, one physician's assistant, and one resident lined up at the foot of my bed. My eyelids opened and slammed shut like there were magnets on the upper and lower lids. I described my back injury once again, from August to yesterday when admitted to the emergency room.

One of the doctors ordered an MRI to get a closer look at the protrusion. I remembered my first MRI after my breast cancer diagnosis, so I felt prepared. Later that afternoon, my friend Shirley came to my room. She was my transporter to take me to the appointment. I welcomed a familiar face and a chance to talk with someone besides medical personnel.

Already cloaked in the appropriate gown, I waited for my turn in the thumping MRI machine. The frigid room brought shivers to my body, and soon an avalanche of bleached white, warm blankets were wrapped around me. I wondered how many bleached white blankets were used in a 24-hour period. Within a few minutes, the technicians wheeled me into the sterile hospital room. They assisted me as I climbed on to the platform and packed cushions around my head and arms. Stuffed into a straitjacket, my adrenalin spiked, searching for all the cells in my body. The technicians started the machine and the tray I laid on maneuvered its way into a tube. Inside, I opened my eyes and I started screaming "Get me out! Get me out!" They knew immediately I had opened my eyes. "Keep your eyes closed and this will be over in 45 minutes," the MRI technician said.

"No! Take the stuffing away from my head and arms. I promise I will not move," I begged them. "This test is not going to happen if you don't take the stuffing away from my arms and head."

They agreed and removed the padding. Once again, I found myself confined to the tube. I lay still for 45 long minutes listening to pounding, throb-like noises with my eyes closed the entire time. When it was over, they thanked me for lying still. I smiled and replied, "Thank you for taking out the padding."

When the results of the MRI were available, the pack of doctors lined up at the foot of my bed again. The MRI provided a closer look at the herniated disc; a large protrusion crowded the nerve which created the constant and severe pain. Their recommendations: to start a drug called Gabapentin, get a steroid injection, or do nothing and go home and rest. The side effects of Gabapentin were dizziness, drowsiness, memory loss, lack of coordination, unsteadiness, tremors, water retention, and on and on. I chose the steroid injection. The first available appointment was in two days, which meant I had to sit and think about a needle being plunged into my spine for two days.

During my hospital stay, I requested to be taken off the narcotics and only given Tylenol and Ibuprofen. While lying flat on my back for three days, I found relief, until I stood up to go to the bathroom, and the pain returned.

When I wasn't reading a book, I dozed off and on or thought about the way I treated my body. Cancer had forced me to take an honest look at myself and my habits. The journey introduced me to self-love and self-care. It wasn't that I didn't know how to love and care for myself, I just had never made it a priority. Of course, I tried it. I loved myself one day and hated myself for the next three days—you aren't smart enough, pretty enough, strong enough. My emotions spiraled like a kite that lost its wind. Cancer, time away from the grind, and the people who walked by me on my journey helped me recognize the beauty I possessed. Not only the external beauty, but more importantly the internal beauty, the beauty that mattered. Though none of my doctors or therapists confirmed that my cancer or my negative self-talk injured my back, I took responsibility for it. My positive attitude helped me beat cancer, and my poor self-talk afterward forced me to push to the extremes during my exercise program. My body simply wasn't ready for the beating I was giving it. Positive self-talk, a delicate evolution, must be tended to and cared for. The negative self-talk must be redirected the second it floated into my head.

When I wasn't thinking about a needle in my spine, I was lamenting about the girl I used to be. The girl who was strong, the girl who literally made people exhale in pain during exercise classes. There were moments of sorrow, moments that made me think about how I continually pushed past limits physically and mentally. Why was it so important for me run a 5K the same year I finished cancer treatment? Did I need to prove something to myself or others? Was it the need to forget about the imposters sewn onto my chest? Was it the need to forget about all the side effects of chemo and radiation? Was it the need to feel that cancer didn't rob me of my physical and mental acuity? The more I thought, the more depressed I became. There were no answers waiting for me. Instead of running a 5K the same year I finished treatment, I found myself under the care of more doctors for a different ailment. I felt broken.

A transporter arrived around 10 a.m. for my first steroid injection. A needle in my spine sounded dangerous, even life-threatening. I wanted to limp back to the hospital bed and stay there forever. The transporter delivered me to a holding room, and I waited for the physician. When he arrived, I signed on the line to illustrate consent. The form acknowledged that the doctor was not responsible for accidents. Fear rushed throughout my brain, I squashed cancer earlier in the year, and now I wondered if a stupid spinal injection was going to be my demise.

The doctor wheeled me down several hallways apologizing for each bump he rolled over, and when he ran into the wall, I thought it was intentional to see how loudly I would yelp from the pain. He wheeled my bed into a room that seemed darker than it should be for someone to see well enough to plunge a needle into my back. The doctors wore bullet proof vests of some sort. I deduced the vests were probably because of the x-ray machine in the room.

Three doctors hovered around my bed and had me log roll from one bed to the other. As they prepped the area on my back between the fourth and fifth lumbar, my nervousness reminded me of first chemo session. I tried to relax. I should have asked for a chill pill.

The doctor alerted me when he numbed the area on my back and described the procedure. An epidural helped combat inflammation in my back. Each step was explained: first the needle was inserted in the area where the disc was herniated. The radiologist moved the x-ray machine to obtain a lateral view to ensure appropriate needle positioning.

"How are you feeling?" One doctor asked.

"Nervous…okay, I guess," I stammered.

Before the steroids were pushed through the needle, the doctor used a dye to check needle placement. Confident with the positioning of the needle, the steroids flowed from the needle and entered my body.

As the steroids arrived inside my system, pressure inundated my right leg. It felt like someone was blowing up my right leg like a balloon. Oh my God, I'm going to pop! I thought. I grunted and moaned sharing my discomfort hoping they would stop. The doctor reduced the speed of the injection as it traveled towards the herniated disc, but he never stopped. My right foot twitched and I wondered if that was a bad omen.

A few minutes later, the procedure was complete. I log rolled back to another bed and they returned me to the private room pre-injection. Before the doctor left my room, he said, "Everything went exactly as planned. How is your pain level?" I rated my pain at a 5 out of 10, only slightly less than when I went in.

"The injection should start taking effect in a couple of days, but it can take up to two weeks," he said.

The nurse brought me another warm blanket. I felt bad for the person who washed and dried the laundry. I waited for my transporter to take me back to my hospital room. That afternoon, I showered on my own, and the doctors finally released me that evening. Prior to my departure, my physician scheduled an appointment with a spine specialist later in the month.

At home, the cats snuggled around me, purring loudly as I laid in bed for another four days sipping water, reading books, and watching Netflix. Nine straight days on my back and no relief in sight. My thoughts tangled with each other. Each day, trying to love myself—to love my body.

I hobbled back to work the following Monday in survival mode. If I stood, the pain diminished slightly, so I raised my standing desk at work and left it there. I asked my supervisors if I could stand during meetings and of course they obliged. Standing was the only way I survived.

So much had changed in my work environment since this time last year. Corporate hired a marketing genius as my supervisor. She brought new ideas and energy to the department and the building. Intelligent, charismatic, compassionate, and a go-getter, she happily shared her knowledge with me to help better my career with the company.

Our senior living community lost a couple of excellent directors, but they moved on to new opportunities. While I was sad to see them go, I understood their choices and wished them well. We welcomed new faces and continued to enjoy our days at work.

I visited with a physician's assistant at the spine clinic in mid-December. I learned from my chiropractor that the excruciating pain I felt in the right outer part of my ankle was a side effect of the nerve under duress. However, when I circled my lower leg pain on the diagram, at the spine clinic, he looked at me and said "You know you're at the spine clinic right? We work on backs here."

True to my nature, I was caught off guard with his remark and choice words parked themselves at the end of my tongue. I learned over time that this character flaw of never saying what was on my mind was a good thing. If I pressed down on the pedal and gave those words gas, I would have been kicked out of the spine center and banned from the clinic.

He reminded me I still had two days left for the steroid injection to take effect. So far, I had zero relief. The PA at the spine clinic said my next option would be surgery where they would cut into my back, remove bone, and take out the protrusion. That devastated me. To a non-medical professional like me, this sounded like a dangerous procedure and should be the last-ditch effort.

The PA said I could try this illustrious Gabapentin or get another injection. I asked about physical therapy because I abhorred the thought of any more drugs introduced to my system. I feared the Red Devil may still be roiling around deep inside me even after a year. No more drugs—Nancy Regan would be proud.

"I can schedule you an appointment with the physical therapist to see if he can help you, or you can try another injection and have the doctor use a different angle to attack the disc protrusion," he said.

"I would be open to another injection and physical therapy." The thought of another injection terrified me but living with severe back pain terrified me even more. My life had been altered with this injury more so than cancer—no running, hardly any walking, no weight training, no yoga, nothing. Even my sex life suffered with a back injury. For a woman, wife, and athlete, this was torture!

The following day, I went to my lymphedema PT appointment. She said the physical therapist I was scheduled to meet with was top-notch—one of the best of the best in terms of back injuries. She was hopeful, and that was all I needed.

About six weeks after my first steroid injection, I returned to the clinic for injection number two. The doctor described the different needle angle and appeared hopeful that I would have relief. I was excited at the thought of putting my own socks and shoes on for a change. His partner for the procedure, a female nurse, held my hand and comforted me when I moaned and groaned during the procedure. The small pinch of the needle, and the pressure in my leg came and went swiftly. He prescribed relaxation for the entire day to ensure the steroid remained in the appropriate location. By now, resting came easily to me. My body must have been punishing me for all those years of brutal workouts and little rest. I was making up for lost time.

Nicole L. Czarnomski

A week after my second injection, still no relief in sight, I met with the new PT, the back specialist. I waited for more than a month to see this doctor, suffering day in day out, crawling out of bed each day hoping for relief. I experienced piercing and searing pain from my lower back to my ankle unless I laid flat on my back. Even while standing, the leg pain was excruciating. As time passed, I stopped engaging in activities with friends, went on fewer dates with my husband, and exercise was at a complete stand-still. The pain was unbearable. It had been two months since I had broken a sweat—minus any hot flashes. At least while I was going through treatments for my cancer, I could still participate in activities I enjoyed.

Twenty-two minutes. The most colossal waste of time I had ever experienced. That was how long my appointment with the physical therapist lasted. His opening remarks, "It's very important to maintain a healthy back. You should complete cardio exercises at least five times a week for 30 minutes. You also need to avoid being overweight." Again, grateful for my inability to speak when caught off guard, it saved me from screaming at him and getting kicked out of the clinic. At this point, my weight dropped below 150 again, and I wanted to tell him to call my plastic surgeon who told me I was too thin to create anything larger than an A-cup. And, how the hell was I supposed to exercise when I could barely walk? Jerk.

This doctor looked me straight in the face and said, "We really want to dodge the surgery bullet, so let's try to keep you away from the surgeon. This procedure requires bone removal, and studies have shown that after five years the patient is usually worse off." This joker literally gave me a DVD, some paperwork, three stretches (the same ones my other physical therapist gave me) and wished me good luck. I felt completely hopeless.

201

I met with my oncologist the following week for my one-year post-chemo check-up. He read about my hospital stay in the notes in my online portal.

"I'm sorry to hear about your back. You've been through so much already. I'm glad it's only a disc and not anything worse," he said. Then he shared his experience with a herniated disc. His happened while he was finishing his residency and taking final exams. "It couldn't have happened at a more inopportune time. I had emergency surgery because the disc ruptured and caused leg pain, weakness, and numbness." He concluded with a success story. "I felt so much better after surgery. And now, my back is strong and healthy." I thanked him for sharing the positive results of his surgery.

As he completed my breast exam, I waited for him to comment on my radiation damaged, grapefruit-like right breast. The poor girl had risen toward my chin and to the right towards my armpit about one centimeter each way. I didn't think this shift could be detected by the naked eye, but truthfully, I didn't know. It looked okay in the mirror, and when I asked Adlai, I received the same response he gave me when I asked if my jeans made me look fat, "Oh, it's time to fight?"

Sometimes when I hugged people I wondered if they could feel the less than squishy right breast attached to my chest like an afterthought. As my oncologist pressed into my right breast scanning for lumps, I couldn't take it anymore. "Radiation wasn't kind to me. Righty isn't super sexy." I realized what I just said while my oncologist searched for lumps. "I mean for my husband. My boobs aren't what they used to be." He continued to probe, concentrating to make sure he didn't miss anything. I appreciated his thorough investigation, but I waited impatiently for a response.

"Nicole, it may feel uncomfortable, but these are cosmetic and minor issues. If having a firm breast bothers you, it can be fixed. I know the lack of sensation is probably frustrating, but you are a healthy

young woman, and everything looks good today." Though I wanted
him to pull a rabbit out of his hat and apply nipples to my breasts that
could sense cold and stimulation like their predecessor, I took his
words to heart, and practiced being happy and free of cancer.

After I was given a clean bill of health during my one-year
post-chemo exam, we discussed the Tamoxifen pill and hot flashes.
"The hot flashes don't bother me too much, especially during the
winter. I actually welcome the warmth each hot flash brought to me this
season," I said. I mentioned some spotting but nothing severe. I told
him I was no longer having periods.

"Did you receive any information from the insurance company
regarding your test for the Tamoxifen?" he asked.

"Yes, they denied my claim even with your letter and
documentation to support your request for this test," I said.

He shook his head in disgust and apologized wishing it would
have turned out differently. At this point, I couldn't care less about the
insurance company denying my appeal. I just wanted my life back. I
wanted to be able to participate in activities of daily living. He wished
me good luck with my back pain, and I took his words to heart, and
practiced being happy and cancer-free.

Almost one month had passed since my second steroid
injection. I found myself standing at my desk, standing in meetings,
avoiding exercise like a cat avoiding water, and popping copious
amounts of Tylenol and Ibuprofen—it's a shame I didn't purchase
stock in one of these drug companies, I'd be a wealthy woman. I had
reached the end of the line. I met with a spine surgeon in early February
2019, less than one year after the end of my cancer treatments. I was

terrified the surgeon was going to take out an entire vertebra, leaving me two inches shorter.

The spine surgeon's office was in the same building where I had my chemo treatments. I hoped PTSD would leave me alone that day. Adlai and I went to this appointment together. There weren't many things we did apart these days. I loved him more deeply than I had ever loved anyone. He made it easy to love him with his kind and gentle nature. He stood by me through one of the most difficult challenges of my life. He loved me when the imposters arrived on my chest. He loved me when I was hairless. He loved me at my weakest, when he had to work a full-time job, and then return home each evening to care for me and take care of the daily chores. He loved me when I lost weight, and when I gained it all back. He saw past my imperfections and loved me anyway. He brought laughter into my life after every downward spiral. I was so grateful to have him by my side for another long journey.

My doctor arrived in my room dressed in hospital scrubs. It was customary to see my physicians dressed in suits, so I was shocked to see him dressed so casually. I wondered if he had already cut on someone that morning. I secretly wished it would have been me on the operating table. Then I remembered he may have to remove my vertebrae. He tested my strength, or in my case, weakness, the way every other doctor had done before him. He explained the procedure—a lumbar discectomy. I tried to remember his exact words, but it was tough to understand the medical terminology, and even more difficult to believe a doctor could do all this work in such a small area—a two-centimeter canal.

Essentially, an incision would be made, the "roof" removed (hemilaminectomy), the canal or bone that housed the nerve, would be carved out (foraminotomy), and the herniated part of the disc removed (microdiscectomy). There was no need for a bone fusion. And of course, he wasn't going to remove my vertebrae. He reassured me the procedure was minimally invasive. The incision would be located along the spine and span a couple of inches. He could see the fear on my face.

"The spinal cord ends much higher up, so there's no chance of spinal cord injury." (No, I didn't pay attention in high school or college biology, so I didn't know the spinal cord ended higher than my L4/L5 herniated disc.) The recovery time would span six weeks. "I recommend the entire six weeks even if you are feeling better. It's imperative you follow BLT. No bending, lifting more than 10 pounds, or twisting. If you do too much, it will cause more damage, and the surgery will be for naught."

He went on to explain the remainder of the procedure. "The incision is sewn together with a few nylon sutures and glue. Many people can leave the same day." I was shocked. Out-patient spine surgery? Still somewhat terrifying, same day surgery did relieve some of my stress. Once I agreed to this treatment, I had to wait another month before the surgeon had an opening. Adlai asked if he had time to do the procedure that day. The surgeon looked at us like we were ignorant. He didn't even crack a smile. I guessed he didn't appreciate the joke.

He had a slot the following Monday, but the insurance company would need to review the case before allowing me to have the procedure. The review could take two weeks! I left the surgeon's office on that frigid February day with hope. Another salesperson. I didn't realize how many health care workers had to sell their specialty, although this doctor didn't have much selling to do. I wanted that damn herniated disc to vacate the premises. One other thing I discovered in talking to him, he believed a cyst may have grown on the herniated portion of the disc making the canal even smaller. The cyst wasn't anything to be concerned about, it was simply putting more pressure on the nerve.

When Adlai and I returned home, we found YouTube videos of the surgery. It looked easy. A small fluoroscope is inserted so the surgeon can see inside. A small amount of lamina or bone that forms the backside of the spinal canal is removed to access the canal. Using a nerve retractor, the surgeon gently moves the nerve out of the way to access the herniated disc. The herniated portion of the disc is removed clearing the area which will allow room for the nerve root. Just like the doctor said. Easy.

I waited the agonizing four weeks like it was Groundhog Day again, just like my radiation treatments but with very different symptoms. I woke up every morning with a shot of pain from my low back through my glute and hip and down to my ankle. I continued working full-time, standing at meetings, at my desk, and eating my lunch. I slogged through the days feeling like the surgery date would never arrive.

My anxiety level peaked and despite the pain, I wondered if I had made the right choice. I was trying to focus on writing and finishing this book, but my head and heart weren't in it. I stopped journaling, and I stopped sending love to my poor herniated disc. I was frustrated, tired, and ready to find relief. I wished someone would have told me to take it easy after my cancer treatments. I wished there would have been an exercise program for women who had recently finished treatments. A program that was slow and steady and helped me build strength and endurance. Maybe then I wouldn't have injured my back.

Occasionally, my back would feel better, until I bent over, tried to put on my socks, or I sneezed too hard. Then pain returned immediately. One Sunday morning while chatting with my friend Beverly, she said she could sense the tension in my body. My voice strained and my body writhed with anxiety. She peeled back my emotions like the layer of an onion when we started to discuss the progress of my book, or lack of progress.

"First, you need to stop beating yourself up over not writing." I was stunned listening to her. I was at it again, trying to hold myself accountable in a time that didn't warrant any scolding. "You can't finish your book when you have an entire chapter that hasn't even happened yet. Once you are through this phase [back surgery] you are going to have the time and energy to focus on writing. Now is not the time. You are in survival mode." Beverly was one of those friends who listened intently to everything I said, analyzed it, and spit it back out in recommendation form before I even ended my sentence.

She was right. After my surgery, I would have the time to write. It angered me that I had to be recovering from yet another ailment, but I was grateful to have the time to heal so I could focus on writing too. Not only could I use the time to write, but I could focus on self-care again—meditation, walking, reading.

# Back Surgery

My parents arrived the day before my surgery. It was March, and we still hadn't celebrated Christmas, so when they arrived, we gathered around our home-made wooden tree wrapped in tinsel and lights. We opened our gifts and talked about the weather. Normally, I saved weather chit chat for people I don't know well or ones I wanted to know, but we had just survived the snowiest February on record. There was upwards of 50 inches of snow that month. Snow mounds were everywhere; it was literally piled to the top of our mailbox.

I was starting to feel bad for my family. First cancer and now back surgery. I don't make anything easy, I thought to myself after we were finished opening gifts. I was grateful to have my parents by my side once again to make it through another difficult journey. I was glad they were there for my husband too. Mr. Fix It couldn't fix any of my ailments. It was like my body poked fun at him, "Haha, bet you thought your mechanical aptitude was off the charts, well, you can't fix me."

That night, I followed orders and created a bubble around myself for yet another surgery. Once again, I cleaned with anti-bacterial soap, but this time the kitties weren't kicked out of my bed— shhhh, don't tell the surgeon.

The following morning, we arrived at the hospital at 9:45 a.m. I exited the car and pain shot through my leg and took my breath away. I wanted to cuss. I wanted to scream. But that day, I didn't have to. Relief was close by.

When we entered the clinic, it was quieter than a morgue, halls void of people. As we navigated through the maze, we turned a corner and finally, life. There was a small coffee shop with a few people waiting in line for their morning cup of coffee. I was envious. I wanted coffee as badly as I wanted my back to be healed. Mornings were my least favorite time of day. They always have been, but today, I was acutely aware of how tired I was. Four months of constant, nagging pain and now the realization that I was going under the knife again made me want to crawl up in a little ball and go back to bed.

When I was kid, I hated mornings as much I hate them now. In my younger years, mom and dad called me their little turtle. They would call out my name every morning trying to oust me from my bed. I don't remember how many times they hollered every morning, but when I finally made it out of bed, I laid on the floor in the hallway with my knees tucked under my chest and a blanket over my body. Not only did I look like a turtle hiding in its shell, but I moved at a turtle's pace.

When I was older, my brother always got to ride shot gun when mom took us to school, because I was still in the house trying to get ready. Every morning, I would hear that same customary honk of the horn letting me know we were running late. And then in high school, it was worse, I earned many tardy slips after I started driving myself to school. I'd leave home late and had to park at least a half a mile away which didn't leave me enough time to make the first bell.

The hallways at the hospital were endless. We searched for the blue sign trying to follow the arrows to the admissions desk. Honestly, I thought we were going to be late to my surgery—par for the course if you schedule something in the morning for me.

The walls were white and lined with brightly colored artwork. I wanted to stop and admire the art with a warm cup of coffee, dissecting it like I did in my college art history classes. It occurred to me that many of the patients don't have time or energy to stop and dissect the work; that was for family members. I suddenly felt an ounce of jealousy. Jealous that my parents could drink coffee and discuss the texture, the color, and the positive and negative space each work of art possessed.

In the admissions area, I was swiftly checked in and offered a seat in the waiting area. I don't think we waited five minutes before a short man who barely spoke English called my first name and then butchered my last name. Growing up with a difficult last name, Heidbreder, and then marrying into another tough name made me numb to the incorrect pronunciations.

He called another man's name and ushered both families down the corridor into the older part of the building. I felt like I was in the psych ward of a hospital that had been around for hundreds of years. The doorways had thick crown molding around the edges and the floors were old tile floors from at least the 50s. As we walked down the hallway, I noticed each room had space for two, and all I could think was, oh my God I am roommates with a man. How am I going to change?

When we arrived at my room, the name on the door had another woman's name. Whew, I dodged a bullet. The nice gentleman who butchered my last name led me into the room and told me to change, even my undergarments. Behind the curtain in my room, my mom waited with me and helped me out of my clothes. Within minutes a nurse arrived to ask questions and take my vitals. My blood pressure was high that morning. It was hovering around 115 over 70. My eyes were like saucers, and I told the nurse that was bad, really bad. She smiled and said, "No that's about normal." I argued with her telling her my blood pressure was usually in the low 90s over low 60s. She smiled again. "Pain and stress are most likely elevating your blood pressure this morning. You have nothing to worry about," she said.

While she was taking my temperature, another man came in who was dressed in hospital scrubs. He looked exactly like the Hollywood movie star, Zach Galifianakis, with corkscrew curls in his hair. While Zach was puncturing my hand, they banded my right wrist with a pink DO NOT TOUCH label. I squirmed and scrunched my face

Nicole L. Czarnomski

as he put the catheter in my hand. "Are you done? Is it in?" I
questioned like a frightened five-year-old girl. He looked at me like I
was a wimp. Okay, so I was a big wimp. Just give me the chill out
medications, I thought to myself. Ten minutes later, they were ready,
no horsing around, no drawing diagrams, no needle localizations, just
here we go. I log rolled onto a gurney, and I was taken to the next
holding cell, my family following behind my wheeled bed. They were
directed to a waiting area, and I was whisked away to a newer part of
the building. Thank goodness. The old ward gave me a bad feeling. I
feared a thunderstorm might happen and a bolt of lightning may hit the
building and the power would go out during surgery leaving me
stranded, my incision wide open, tools stuck in my back while doctors
head lamps were the only thing lighting up the room.

My holding cell was small and dark, perfect for a bear going
into hibernation mode. The nurse tried to scan my wrist band, but it
wasn't working. Her laugh bellowed outside of my room and down the
hall. She looked at me when the other nurse arrived and said, "Do you
mind if I cuss?"

I looked at her with a straight face and said, "Lady, if you
dropped the F-Bomb right now, I would be really happy!" And then I
smiled and remembered the Happiness book and wished I could add a
page about the F-bomb being happiness.

"Well, this fucking thing isn't scanning and now I don't know
what to do!" She exclaimed. All three of us had a good laugh.
Whatever it was they were doing finally worked and they left me alone
in the small cave.

A couple more doctors entered my room. First an
anesthesiologist, who I begged for anti-nausea medications in my
cocktail. He asked if I'd like the scopolamine patch. "Yes!" I said
emphatically. "And use everything you can in my cocktail." I felt like I

211

was at a bar back in college ordering shots for my friends, "Slippery Nipples, JagerBombs, and Jell-o shots for everyone!"

The next doctor that arrived in my holding cell was a fellow, which I later found out was someone going through the Mayo graduate school program. He was fast-tracked, so in other words a really smart dude. He said he would be helping my surgeon during the procedure. Shortly after I was prepped in the holding cell, I was wheeled away by another strange person, the gurney pusher. I asked if he was my nurse, and he said no. Another doctor? No. So, the gurney pusher. I wondered if he had to push dead people. I shivered at the thought, and quickly pushed that out of my head.

I was wheeled into a massive room with huge lights suspended from the ceiling. The lights looked like something found on a spaceship. The overhead lights were large circular saucers, inside the saucers there were mini lights. On a shelf along the far wall, tools and gadgets were spread out awaiting my surgery. At this point I couldn't understand why I hadn't been drugged yet. "Oh my God, Oh my God, OH MY GOD! What is this place?"

"Relax, this is the operating room, and we'll prep you for surgery right here."

I squeezed my eyes shut so nothing could seep in between my eyelids. "What is this?! I don't like this!" I was talking like I had no idea what was going on—like I had been kidnapped and shoved in a basement. The care team witnessed my full-on panic attack, and suddenly, lights out. I don't remember anything after that moment.

I woke up in a beautiful private room on the eighth floor with my family waiting for me. I felt amazing! It was a scary yet refreshing feeling. Lying in bed after being sliced open, bone removed, nerves pushed aside and then stitched back together, I felt nothing. I was laying on my back not a care in the world. My one question, why was I in the private room and not the old ward? As usual, my blood pressure dropped. Dropped to the low 80s over low 50s. That always concerned the nurses. I was being monitored, and they were keeping me overnight.

Thank goodness, I thought to myself. I don't want my family taking care of me. What if something goes wrong? I lived 30 minutes away. We'd have to drive back in the middle of the night.

Much of the night was interrupted by polite nurses taking my vitals and getting me up to go to the bathroom. They really wanted me to fart too. They kept asking, "Did you pass gas?" I always replied, "No," disappointing them each time. I thought about asking for Chipotle, extra beans.

My first two nurses were male. They offered to help me wipe when I was finished peeing. My response, "No, I'm not gonna make you do that." Both male nurses were polite and professional.

"That's my job. I am paid to wipe you," both said. I declined their help, and they gave me privacy.

The following morning, I waited for the drugs to wear off, but sleep was winning the battle. I couldn't keep my eyes open. Doctors arrived, asked how I was feeling, while I struggled to form sentences. Apparently, my blood pressure was asleep too. Each nurse would check it and then ask to take it again. I smiled and said with a dazed looked on my face, "I'm great. Don't worry it's always low."

"Oh, 82 over 50. That is a little low." But it concerned them more than it concerned me.

The physical therapist arrived to get me up and walking. I could barely make it around the small nurse's station using a walker. I was exhausted, lightheaded. I needed to rest. I sat in a chair in the nurse's station after walking about 20 feet. When I wasn't lightheaded anymore, I stood and walked back to my room, eager to sleep.

My family arrived late morning thinking I would be ready to go. After waiting a couple of hours and watching me sleep, my family went grocery shopping, took everything home, and returned mid-afternoon. I had barely moved since they left. I couldn't shake the overwhelming exhaustion. If I wanted out of the hospital, I was going to have to walk and make it look good. I forced myself to get up and walk around the nurse's station with my old lady walker. I was as rickety as an old fence post standing there. As I trudged around the eighth floor, the physical therapist said she would ask the doctor for a prescription for a walker.

Prescription for a walker! No! Hell No! I was not leaving this joint with a walker. I had a cane at home and could use it to get around. Four simple words, prescription for a walker, got me up and walking again and again. Tiny little steps, like I was an infant learning to walk. Those baby steps were all I could manage for over a week.

By 4:30 that afternoon, I wondered if I was ever going to get out of the hospital. I almost wanted to stay because I didn't feel strong enough to walk. But I decided I could do it and urged the nurses to hurry up with the discharge paperwork.

The last nurse I was assigned must have been right out of school. She really pissed me off. I wanted them to take my blood pressure now to see how high it soared. She came in with documents for my discharge and reviewed the dos and don'ts post-surgery. No sitting longer than 20 minutes. I flipped. "You've had me sitting in a chair for two hours!" I shrieked.

Nicole L. Czarnomski

"Oh, it's okay, this is a generic form. You're fine." She continued reviewing the rules, but she was all over the place. Scanning the top, jumping to the bottom with her shifty eyes, do this, no that's fine, do that, oh no, that's fine too.

I asked for a number to call if something went wrong. "If something goes wrong..." her sentence trailed off and she looked at me like I was the healthiest person in the world who didn't just have back surgery. "Um, I don't know. Lemme check."

When she returned, she said, "Just call this number. It's this floor."

"Okay, what's the on-call number?" I asked.

"Just call this one."

"No, I want the on-call number for the surgeon on duty."

"Um, I don't know. Lemme check."

I was seething. If I was a wild animal, I would have been foaming at the mouth.

When she left my room again, I bolted out of bed, forgetting I had finished surgery just yesterday. "What is going on?" I asked as nerve pain shot through my ankle. "Can I sit for more than 20 minutes?"

The group of nurses at the nurse station looked at me like I was a scared cat up a tree because I was a scared cat up a tree. They reassured me that sitting was fine, but I needed to be up moving around often. They recommended that I walk farther and farther each day. I wondered what that meant. How far? If I walked too far, could that cause damage? I was still uncomfortable with the thought of going home that afternoon, but they finally cut me loose. Perhaps getting the

215

newbie nurse to discuss my discharge was what I needed to get angry and to get my blood pressure to rise. We picked up the narcotic prescriptions and left the hospital around 5 p.m.

The car ride home was miserable. The narcotics had worn off and I was only taking Tylenol. My choice, and not a good one, I might add. Every bump, pothole, and crack delivered a shot of pain into my back. "Give me the drugs!" I took one of the Tramadol pills so I could survive the ride home. The next couple of days were a blur. My parents and my husband bustled around the house, cleaning, making food, and running errands.

At first, I walked around the house, trying to will my back into healing quickly. I walked around the house on an hourly basis, trying not to sit too long for fear of messing everything up. My old warrior-like personality felt kicked, beaten, and given the big F-U. I couldn't understand where the fear was coming from. I beat cancer for goodness sakes. Why was I so upset and freaked out about my back not healing correctly? I needed to change my attitude. Somewhere along the way, my strength had been taken away, stolen, and replaced by fear and self-loathing. I had to find my will, my desire to want to be whole again, and to trust my surgeon and spine care team as much as I trusted my oncologist and my cancer care team.

My parents left that following Monday, and I spent the next few days wallowing in fear. My mind was filled with terrifying thoughts of having to go back into surgery and to have more of my disc removed. My foot tingled. Oh no! I ruined it, the narrator in my head shouted me! My ankle bone still hurts. Oh no! I ruined it! I sat too long. I walked too far. I didn't walk far enough.

Three days after my parents left, I put the kibosh on the pity party. I had had enough of myself. I found guided meditation videos for healing the body. I journaled, I walked, I ate, I rested, I meditated, I read books, I slept. I dug myself out of the pit of despair and started functioning on a higher frequency. My confidence returned, I was healing, and I treated my body like I did during cancer treatments. I was kind and loving and patient.

At my two-week check-up, my nurse said the lower leg pain was most likely going to continue for up to six months. Apparently, nerves healed slower than anything else in the body. She also said it was time to remove the stitches in my back. I shuddered to think my incision was ready to have the stitches removed, but she reassured me everything was fine.

"If we don't take them out there could be permanent scarring," she said. The two-and-a-half-inch incision was not a pretty sight. It looked like Hannibal Lecter had used a quarter inch thick piece of leather and sewed five stitches over the incision in the shape of an X. It looked hideous. The stitches were bad enough, but the glue over the stitches created a pooch at the top of the wound. It was like the doctor didn't account for gravity when he closed the incision, me still lying flat on my back.

When my surgeon arrived, his straight face and serious demeanor annoyed me. He was nothing like my oncologist who was gregarious, jovial, and genuinely interested in my well-being. My gut said, this guy hates me. He never cracked a smile, not even when I clapped my hands together to celebrate my lengthy walk the day before. "3000 steps!" I beamed.

He asked if I wanted to see the photo of the herniated portion of my disc that he removed. I was elated. "Yes, I want to see the little monster!" I exclaimed. I wanted to feel validated, I wanted to know why I had been suffering for so long.

His nurse pulled up the two images on the computer. One was the canal where the herniated disc was located, and the other picture was the portion they removed. Both pictures made me cringe. "Oh God, that's disgusting," I said scrunching my face.

The picture with the gel-filled nucleus was sitting on a blue tissue. There was some type of measuring device along the bottom and right side. The units were in centimeters. He said he removed a chunk about one centimeter by one and a half centimeters. He continued by saying this may appear very small, but the canal it shared with my nerve was two centimeters. I was shocked and validated—not that I needed to be. But I wanted to make sure if there were any naysayers thinking I was faking it, ha, the pain was real and now I knew why.

He tested my leg strength and suggested I stretch my hamstrings. Hamstrings become less flexible and tight with back injuries. He was right, I couldn't sit and extend either leg to a straight position. He proceeded to tell me to be very cautious with the BLT rule. No bending, lifting more than ten pounds, or twisting for four more weeks. "At six weeks, we'll schedule you for imaging and review your status. Then, you can begin physical therapy to strengthen your stomach and back." Happy with my results, I returned home to write, read, rest, walk, eat, meditate, and sleep. I was once again on the road to recovery.

Nicole L. Czarnomski

# I'm a Survivor

It's my one-year anniversary! One-year since my last radiation treatment. It was difficult to believe all that time had already passed. I arrived at my physical therapy appointment—my breast cancer PT. We discussed my progress. While I still had a slightly misplaced boob (not as bad as it was one year ago) that felt like a grapefruit, my mobility had improved. Jenny had pushed and pulled on the taut cording in my armpit for over a year. I could finally see the progress.

We discussed options for creating a softer, squishy boob. She said the clinic had hired a new plastic surgeon who was making great strides in breast reconstruction. Although going under the knife at this point sounded dreadful (only four weeks since my back surgery), at least there were options for me in the future.

To celebrate my victory over cancer, Adlai and I shared a drink and a meal at Twig's, the same place we went one year ago to celebrate my final radiation treatment. Still a mystery as to where time went, we sat across from each other smiling and gazing into each other's eyes. At first, I didn't know what to say, but when our drinks arrived, we raised our glasses, and at that moment a flood of memories passed through my brain. I was grateful to have my toenails and fingernails healthy again. My hair was the cutest it had ever been, and each time I walked into the salon to have it trimmed, I always smiled and said, "Let's keep it short." The eyebrows and eyelashes had returned, and I no longer looked "sick." I continued to wear fun earrings because they stood out against my short hair, and I loved it! My heart rate had slowed down since I was no longer taking steroids. Eighty beats per minute. Not great, but at least my chest didn't feel like a ticking time bomb. The minor chest pains I had during chemo stopped. I like to think the chest pains were my heart healing from the negativity in my past. The scars across my nippleless chest had faded, and while I miss the sensations I used to have, I had accepted this as my new normal and would continue learning to love the new me. The post-cancer me. Thankfully, the Tamoxifen pill that forced me into menopause did not hinder our sex life; we are a happy and healthy couple in so many ways. As we touched our glasses together during that toast, I thanked Adlai for his support, for being so strong, for working so hard at his job to keep food on the table, a roof over our heads, and clothing on our backs. My eyes full of the sincerest adoration for any human being, I toasted, "Cheers for what's to come!"

I'm not the girl I used to be. My abilities are never going to be the same. Dealing with physical ailments didn't break me, I was already broken. Instead, these monumental battles put me back together. I love to take walks. I love the changing of the seasons, the lush green in the summer and the fiery red and ochre leaves of fall. I love to watch the snow blanket my surroundings and the shy raindrops cling to the windows. I love the warm sunshine on my pale, freckled skin and the gnarly gruff sounds of a spring thunderstorm. I love each passing day. I love so many aspects of life and so many people, but most importantly, I love me and my simple imperfections, like the dimple on my cheek when I smile.

# Acknowledgements

Writing about my cancer journey started as a cathartic way to manage fear and celebrate milestones. I jokingly gave it the title "Journey of My Jugs," and it helped me process my decisions and later felt like a great way of sharing with others. As I continued the process, I had to relive deeply painful experiences over and over as I edited this book. I could not have written or finished this book without the love and support of so many people just like I would have never survived my cancer journey without the help of others.

To my husband, who walked beside me through some of the darkest days of my life. You carried me over many hurdles all while supporting us financially. You made me laugh when all my smiles were too tired and worn out. Adlai, I love you and thank you from the bottom of my heart.

To my mother, my greatest cheerleader. Thank you for the grace you have given me to walk down many difficult paths, but mostly my cancer journey. Without your influence I would not have made it through with a positive attitude and grace under duress.

Dad your unending jokes made each step a little easier and a little funnier. You took my mind off being broken and helped me laugh again.

To my brother: it took cancer to get you to come and see me! Just kidding little brother. Having you here twice in one year was pretty damn special, and I hope you know just how much I love being your sis.

Angie, thank you for being a rock for my mom to rely on. I appreciate it more than you will ever know.

Sarah, you never missed a chemo treatment. You brought the biggest smile and all the love I needed to survive a grueling journey. And your home cooked meals were a huge help for both Adlai and myself. I'm lucky to know such a great cook!

Dear, sweet Ann, I love all the books you gave me to read to pass the time. Your willingness to help me push this book over the finish line is truly appreciated. Thank you so much for your thoughtful comments.

Katie, you are my girl! You got me the biggest and best room at the end of the hall so I could have a somewhat peaceful evening after my surgery. I can't express how much I appreciate your opinion early on and recommending the "Dream Team."

My dear Kellie, you are a shining star. Thank you for bringing your newborn baby to my pre-chemo party. She brought me hope that night and reminded me that life goes on even through difficult periods of time. And, my radiation team loved your cute cake pops!

Dearest Kathy, thank you for taking walks with me and listening to me when I needed it most. You also make damn good quiche by the way.

To Beverly, I want to express my sincerest gratitude. You spent countless hours on the phone with me helping me through rough patches and celebrating milestones from afar. Your help with final edits was greatly appreciated.

To Denise, my yoga instructor who came to visit me at all my chemo appointments. Your calming and quiet voice wrapped me in love. Your beautiful smile was always a welcome sight. Thank you for holding space for me.

Allison Roe your diligence and sensitivity to editing this book are appreciated more than you will ever know. You sent me comforting thoughts when I felt like an imposter and praised me and reminded me that I just wrote a BOOK!

To my sweet, caring friends and family, Carrie, Tami, Jyll, Marcia, Liz, Derek and Lori, Chuck and Stefani, Corey, and Brittney, thank you for your encouragement, kindness, and generosity. Each one of you helped me along my journey, and I am forever grateful.

Laura Drew you are a superstar! You listened to what I wanted and developed an absolutely stunning book cover.

Beth Anderson, thank you for making my book Kindle and print-on-demand ready.

To my co-workers, thank you for picking up the slack while I was gone. I will always be grateful to you. And to my managers, thank you for your patience as I fought for my life.

And to my cancer care team at both clinics. You didn't always bring me the news I wanted to hear, but in the end, you brought me the life I wanted to live.

# Resources

## Yoga on YouTube

Yoga with Adrienne

Yoga Shala

Yoga by Candace

Yoga with Kassandra

## Meditation on YouTube

Great Meditation

Psyche Truth

The Honest Guys

Stay Well

## Books

Happiness Is… 500 Things to be Happy About
 By Lisa Swerling and Ralph Lazar

The Artist's Way
 By Julia Cameron

The Vein of Gold
 By Julia Cameron

Walking in This World
 By Julia Cameron

Everyday Gratitude: Inspiration for Living Life as a Gift